"I'm thrilled with this book! I spent much of my career trying unsuccessfully to convince the field of psychiatry that IFS was effective with difficult to treat conditions like OCD. Melissa Mose is an OCD specialist who has a depth of knowledge about and experience with the condition. She knows the pluses and minuses of the traditional exposure approach, and, in this well-written book, she deftly combines elements of exposure with a thorough understanding of IFS. She provides ample case examples complete with transcribed dialogues and extensive details in terms of how to implement her approach. I believe this represents a breakthrough in the treatment of OCD and Melissa exhibits such mastery that I suspect many OCD specialists will be tempted to try it out."

Dick Schwartz, PhD, *developer of the IFS model and adjunct faculty member in the Department of Psychiatry Harvard Medical School*

"Melissa Mose's book is a groundbreaking resource for those struggling with OCD. Her integration of Internal Family Systems and traditional exposure techniques offers a fresh, compassionate approach to treatment. It's wonderful to see Melissa exploring the relational aspects that may affect people with OCD not just the symptoms. With rich case examples and practical techniques, this book is a must-read for anyone looking to deepen their understanding of OCD and IFS."

Stuart Ralph, *host of The OCD Stories podcast and co-founder of The Integrative Centre for OCD Therapy*

"Melissa Mose has done it! If you're a therapist, this book is for you. Lost when it comes to OCD? Get this book. Intimately familiar with OCD, but wondering about Internal Family Systems (IFS)? Again, read this! It will help. Specializing in IFS but spinning in circles with clients' obsessive managers, compulsive firefighters, and exiles' energy? Stop spinning, slow down, and read Melissa's clarifying synthesis of present-day best practices for OCD couched in the Internal Family Systems model."

Dan Reed, PhD, LPC, *lead trainer for the Internal Family Systems (IFS) Institute*

"Melissa Mose reframes OCD through the lens of IFS. This transformative fusion weaves in insights on trauma and the complexities that may challenge conventional treatment methods. Through this approach, the path to recovery becomes accessible to individuals who find ERP methods daunting or unsuitable."

Melissa Quinn, MD, *psychiatrist and OCD specialist, maintains a private practice in Los Angeles, and specializes in the treatment of anxiety and obsessive-compulsive disorder*

"Internal Family Systems (IFS) for OCD introduces a contextual, creative, self-compassionate, and experiential route to conceptualization and treatment of the whole person. This book offers one of the clearest and most comprehensive overviews of evidence-based treatments, assessment measures, and a review of similarities and differences between commonly integrated approaches paired with ERP. For this integrative and relational ERP therapist, IFS for OCD feels like a missing puzzle piece that makes space for much deeper work. I am excited about this experiential and relational approach."

Kim Cox, LMFT, *anxiety and OCD and parenting specialist*

"Melissa Mose has written a brilliant book about the treatment of OCD! Her work integrates all the wisdom, compassion, and deep healing of Internal Family Systems (IFS) with the more traditional behavioral exposure and response prevention therapy (ERP) to create a truly new approach to help clients overcome their obsessions and compulsions. This book is packed with practical wisdom, case examples, and techniques that will inspire and guide any therapist who works with OCD. It's a must read!"

Colleen West, LMFT

"As a psychologist with lived experience with OCD, I'm grateful for Melissa's contribution to our field. Deepening our understanding of OCD through the conceptual framework of IFS, integrated with current evidence-based models, and illuminating the dynamic inner world of OCD and related subsystems. Invaluable insight for fostering healing and Self-trust."

Amber Baker, PhD, *clinical psychologist*

"This long-awaited book integrates the benefits of Internal Family Systems (IFS) and exposure and response prevention therapy (ERP) for clients with OCD, and it brings hope to all of us who work with and love them. Melissa Mose aspired to establish a treatment approach that could make recovery possible for individuals who are not able or willing to do traditional ERP, and she succeeded. Melissa is an integrative thinker; she had to be. We are the fortunate recipients of the knowledge she shares culled from her lived experience, determination, compassion, and extraordinary dedication."

Nancy L. Morgan, MS, PhD, *clinical psychologist*

Internal Family Systems Therapy for OCD

Internal Family Systems Therapy for OCD offers a groundbreaking integration of the compassionate, parts-based IFS approach with evidence-based OCD treatments.

This innovative guide introduces IFS for OCD and demonstrates Self-led Exposure and Response Prevention (Self-led ERP), a unique approach that maintains therapeutic effectiveness of treatments that work while enhancing client engagement and facilitating enduring recovery. This approach helps clients develop healing relationships with the protective parts driving the obsessions and compulsions that perpetuate OCD. Through detailed case examples and practical techniques, clinicians learn to help clients access their inherent self-leadership, transform their relationship with uncertainty and fear, and achieve not just symptom reduction but internal balance, harmony, and perspective. This vital resource bridges the gap between relational psychotherapy and behavioral interventions, offering hope for clients who haven't fully responded to conventional treatments.

This invaluable book is essential reading for family therapists and clinical psychologists who are interested in IFS and treat clients with OCD and other anxiety disorders.

Melissa Mose, LMFT, President of OCD Southern California, a non-profit affiliate of the IOCDF, is an OCD specialist and certified IFS therapist.

Internal Family Systems Therapy for OCD
A Clinician's Guide

Melissa Mose

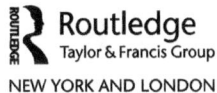

NEW YORK AND LONDON

Designed cover image: Getty Images

First published 2026
by Routledge
605 Third Avenue, New York, NY 10158

and by Routledge
4 Park Square, Milton Park, Abingdon, Oxon, OX14 4RN

Routledge is an imprint of the Taylor & Francis Group, an informa business

© 2026 Melissa Mose

The right of Melissa Mose to be identified as author of this work has been asserted in accordance with sections 77 and 78 of the Copyright, Designs and Patents Act 1988.

All rights reserved. No part of this book may be reprinted or reproduced or utilised in any form or by any electronic, mechanical, or other means, now known or hereafter invented, including photocopying and recording, or in any information storage or retrieval system, without permission in writing from the publishers.

Trademark notice: Product or corporate names may be trademarks or registered trademarks, and are used only for identification and explanation without intent to infringe.

ISBN: 978-1-032-58374-7 (hbk)
ISBN: 978-1-032-58373-0 (pbk)
ISBN: 978-1-003-44981-2 (ebk)

DOI: 10.4324/9781003449812

Typeset in Sabon
by codeMantra

To Claire, whose time in a dark place led me to pursue this path and write this book. You are my inspiration for everything.

Contents

Acknowledgments	*xi*
Foreword by Jeff Szymanski	*xiii*
Foreword by Martha Sweezy	*xvii*
Preface	*xix*
Introduction	1

PART I
Introduction to Internal Family Systems Therapy — 7

1 The Internal Family Systems Approach — 9
2 The Process and Methods of IFS Therapy — 21

PART II
What to Know about OCD — 39

3 An Overview of OCD — 41
4 Assessment and Diagnosis of OCD — 57
5 Evidence-Based Treatment Options for OCD — 69

PART III
The Theory of IFS for OCD — 85

6 An IFS Conceptualization of OCD — 87

7 The OCD Cycle through an IFS Lens	103
8 Why and How IFS Can Be Useful for Clients with OCD	115

PART IV
The Practice of IFS for OCD: Self-led ERP   135

9 IFS-Informed Assessment of OCD	137
10 Stage One: Relating to Protectors and Accessing Self	149
11 Stage Two: Encountering and Unburdening Exiles	169
12 Stage Three: Reconnecting with Protectors	185
Afterword	203
Index	205

Acknowledgments

I first want to express my immense gratitude to Dick Schwartz, both for creating the IFS model and for his willingness to listen to and support my "out of the box" ideas about taking it into new territory. Martha Sweezy and Jeff Szymanski were the intellectual pillars of this project and provided the support without which this book would not exist. Martha's steadfast encouragement—first that I try an IFS training and then to "be brave" about expressing my ideas—and Jeff's consistent guidance—ensuring that my approach remained true to the needs of the OCD community—together helped me find the confidence to stay the course.

Thank you to my primary supporters, my friends and family: to Steve Postell who unwaveringly encouraged me to trust the creative process and to stick with it; to Greg and Sophia Mose, my emotional cornerstones; to Dana Pomfret for camaraderie and laughter; to Suzan Postel for her kindness and support; and to everyone who offered wisdom and moral support, including Toni Cicatello, Pam Pacelli, Mary McCusker, Elliott Beenk, Daryl Ogden, Estee Diamond and Paula Michaels, and Ken McLeod.

I thank all of the friends, colleagues, consultees, and early supporters who have contributed considerably to this book, including Mary Kruger, Mariel Pastor, Dan Reed, Ruth Culver, Colleen West, Nancy Morgan, Marcella Cox, Hanna Soumerai Rei, Bronwyn Shroyer, Mike Heady, Sally Winston, Max Maisel and the gang, Evie Gould, Michelle Witkin, Kim Cox, Kim Rockwell-Evans, Molly Martinez, Natasha Daniels, Christine Izquierdo, Lisa Weiner, Shulamit Widasky, Bob Engel, Yonit Arthur, Amanda Steed, Robert Petrone, and Amber Baker. Thank you to Anibal Henriques and Alexia Rothman, Tammy Sollenberger, Stuart Ralph, Pilar de la Torre and Imma Loret, and Ciara McGriskin and the late Derek Scott for helping me get the work out there. And of course, my heartfelt gratitude to all my clients who were willing to explore and took me with them.

I thank my editors: Marisa Solis, who got me started, as well as Dana Pomfret, Jane Gerhard, and Elizabeth Dougherty for their commitment to clarity. My deep appreciation goes to Ea Macom, whose relentless pursuit of coherence made the arguments sharper and the examples more vivid—and helped me discover what I was really trying to say. Thank you, also, to my Routledge editors, Julia Giordano and Pragati Sharma, for their interest, patience, and support.

And my love to my parents: to Dad, who taught me that it's OK to rock the boat, and to Mom, who taught me how to do it with grace.

Foreword by Jeff Szymanski

Since my days in graduate school, I've been interested in "what works" in therapy. And, I believe in evidence-based practice treatment approaches. I have decades of training and experience using cognitive behavior therapy (CBT), dialectical behavior therapy (DBT), exposure and response prevention (ERP) therapy, and acceptance and commitment therapy (ACT). Effective and impactful psychotherapy is grounded in theory, coherent and accessible to clients, and backed by research. I believe that current treatments for obsessive-compulsive disorder (OCD) can be effective and helpful—even life changing for many. However, there's still room to improve.

One of my primary duties as the executive director of the International OCD Foundation (IOCDF; 2008–2023) was to help protect the OCD community from ineffective treatments. I had learned to be on guard when someone came to me with a "new approach" to therapy having seen so many individuals over the years mired in useless and ineffective treatments for their OCD. However, I was curious when Melissa asked me to help consult on this book. Knowing her to be an excellent ERP therapist she had my attention.

I was not familiar with Internal Family Systems (IFS) therapy, but as Melissa walked me through the basic tenets of IFS therapy for OCD (covered here in Part I), I quickly had a few realizations. First, there was something very resonant about the idea that we all have a "multiplicity" inside us. Everyone uses phrases like "This part of me wants this, but this other part of me wants that." Second, IFS for OCD actually looked a lot like exposure therapy! (Melissa covers exposure in therapy Part II.) From my perspective, as a therapeutic mechanism, engaging in "exposure" means adopting a curious, open, and willing stance while moving toward something that one typically moves away from, with the goal of learning something new. While traditional ERP is primarily focused on moving toward external stimuli, IFS seems to emphasize different ways to approach difficult internal stimuli. A core concept in ACT as well.

Third, I was struck by the centrality of the concept of "Self" in the IFS model. Although I had trained in multiple therapy approaches that acknowledged the importance of "self" (e.g., Albert Bandura's model of self-efficacy), it never seems to be the main focus of treatment. Reflecting on my experience at the OCD Institute at Harvard Medical School's McLean Hospital, working with clients whose symptoms were too severe for outpatient care, I remembered seeing an interesting pattern in many of the clients I was working with. A client who was making progress would suddenly stall or even retreat. "What's going on?" I would ask. The client would reply something along the lines of: "When my symptoms started to go away, I felt like my *self* was disappearing. I didn't know who I was without my symptoms."

Reflecting more on this, I realized that many times when I begin working with a client with OCD, I have the sense that there's no "self" there—just a cluster of symptoms, worries, and concerns. Everything is in the abstract and the world of possibility, alongside the anguish of chronic suffering. I'm not talking to a Self, but I am talking to someone blindly and desperately in need of "protection." It's like we aren't even having a real conversation. And now, I realize, we aren't. I'm talking to "parts" that are masquerading as Self. When I understand instead that I'm encountering a person's protective "parts" trying to manage a terrible sense of vulnerability while being unaware of Self (all this is covered in Part III), then OCD conversations make more sense. I no longer dismiss a symptom with, "Oh, that's just your OCD talking; ignore it." I now encourage clients with OCD to listen to their parts. "Hey, some part of you needs attention! Let's take time to listen. I bet we'll learn something important. Then we can see what needs to happen." That's the process that Melissa lays out in Part IV. When we listen, it doesn't mean we have to agree. Once a part feels heard, it doesn't gain momentum, it quiets down.

I'm glad I was open to learning from Melissa because now I find myself helping clients access and build Self more directly. If we are going to ask clients to do the hard work of exposure-based therapy, we need to have their buy-in. Their Self—a calm, curious, and compassionate Self—needs to be in the driver seat. For some clients, they come to treatment motivated and on board. They respond extremely well to ERP. They also happen to be quite skillful already and have a good sense of Self. However, many clients do not show up that way. And when they don't, pushing them through ERP exercises feels painful to both them and us. So, for some, IFS may be the initial "way in" they need to get started; for others, it may enhance the work they're already doing in ERP. As therapists, we need more tools to help those who haven't been helped or who have not been helped enough. A 30–50% reduction in symptoms may be a great result for a research grant, but it isn't great when someone is suffering. We need to keep looking for the most effective tools to help those who haven't been helped or have not been helped enough.

As Melissa writes in this book, "The goal of IFS therapy is to help parts find a path to beneficial ways of operating—not to ignore, suppress, control, or otherwise try to change them." Since this statement describes the essence of exposure therapy, I think IFS has something very important to offer the OCD community.

Jeff Szymanski, PhD
Founder and CEO, Getting to the Next Level Consulting, LLC
Clinical Instructor, part-time, Harvard Medical School
Clinical Associate, McLean Hospital
Former Executive Director, International OCD Foundation
Former Director of Psychological Services, OCD Institute, McLean Hospital/Harvard Medical School

Foreword by Martha Sweezy

When Melissa Mose called me several years ago to ask for my thoughts about enrolling in an IFS training, I said what I always say, "IFS transformed my views on everything, not just my practice as a therapist. I think you'll find it interesting and useful." In subsequent conversations, we talked about exposure therapy, which I was familiar with through reading about CBT for post-traumatic stress disorder as a second-stage treatment for clients who had been in DBT groups. I said,

> In my view, everything we do in IFS is exposure, but we do it differently. The part or parts who are afraid are not approaching anything alone. They are literally or figuratively holding hands with a compassionate, powerful, validating internal presence who inspires courage. In the process of approach, we don't override, dismiss, or suppress fear, we help the client access an overarching inner confidence that makes approach possible and, ultimately, rewrites the story that led to a poisoned identity.
> (I am ... *weak, helpless, defective, worthless, unlovable*, and so on.)

Since then, Melissa and I have had many discussions about how to apply IFS with OCD. I've learned from her and vice versa. Melissa wrote this book for the OCD community and together we are writing a book on OCD and IFS for the IFS community. The process has helped us to be better therapists—and we hope the resulting books will do the same for you.

Martha Sweezy, PhD
Assistant Professor, part-time, in Psychiatry, Harvard Medical School

Preface

One December morning in 2010, my normally cheerful third grader woke up gripped by intense, irrational fears, agitation, and despair. Seemingly out of nowhere, she began to ask repetitive questions for hours at a time and started to fear that her favorite foods were poisoned. She became terrified of dying, and dying in irrational ways—for example, if her Legos didn't click into place correctly or if she might accidentally swallow magnets. At first, we didn't understand what was going on with her. I did everything I could think of to reassure her that she would be OK and to relieve her suffering, but it only made things worse. With 15 years of experience as a licensed marriage and family therapist, I thought I should know what to do, but I quickly discovered that none of my education or training had equipped me with the tools to help her.

Over the next few months, my daughter's symptoms and their consequences became more dire. She avoided many of her toys, engaged in repetitive behaviors like going back and forth through doorways, and she did not want to leave my side. She refused to go into her bedroom, stopped using certain words, and balked at wearing particular colors. She wouldn't go into grocery stores, and her food choices became increasingly restricted. Progressively frantic, I researched her condition and sought advice throughout my professional community. After many false starts with therapists suggesting a range of possibilities, a psychologist familiar with OCD confirmed my growing suspicions that my daughter was in its grip. With this diagnosis, we eventually found ourselves at the UCLA Pediatric OCD Intensive Outpatient program, where—to our relief—the clinicians had seen all of this before and knew how to help.

For a month, my daughter, at nine years old, received intensive CBT with ERP for three hours a day, four days a week—treatment that was often excruciating for her. She was instructed to wear the scary colors, write the scary words, and sleep next to a collage of frightening images. She was coached to eat the snacks provided for her even though they had been left unguarded in a room, and she feared that they might be poisoned. And although she hated the therapy, she began to experience dramatic improvement after just three weeks: She stopped actively avoiding many of the things she feared, played with her favorite toys again, and began to eat more regularly. Even though my heart broke as I watched her drag herself through these difficult experiences, I couldn't argue with the results: The treatment was working. As I write this, she is in her final year of college, where she is thriving. Although she will probably always have what she calls "quirks," she is free to live her life as the joyous and funny girl she had been before the day her OCD began.

My daughter's journey was the start of a new education for me. Like many clinicians educated in the early 1990s, I had been trained in psychodynamic theory and family systems therapy. As a licensed marriage and family therapist (LMFT), I worked with adolescents and their families, treating a wide range of issues from substance abuse and eating disorders to educational and learning challenges. I had completed my PhD coursework and was in the process of finishing research for my dissertation when everything changed. Because of my firsthand experience with the transformation that CBT with ERP brought about in my daughter, I became dedicated to learning how to offer that level of healing to others. I put aside my work on attachment theory, went back into training, and studied behavioral therapy at the International OCD Foundation's Behavioral Therapy Training Institute. There, I learned the basics of exposure therapy and why it works. I then joined the staff of an OCD clinic for a year to gain more experience, was mentored by a master clinician, and refocused my private practice. For more than 12 years now, 95% of my clients come to me with main complaints of OCD, anxiety, and related disorders. Over the years, I have continued to use evidence-based exposure therapy with my clients, and I have witnessed its efficacy for most of them.

Still, I am well aware that even when ERP is effective, its partial recovery rate leaves many people struggling with ongoing limitations throughout their lives. In addition, some people do not respond to ERP at all, and others cannot or will not participate. Many clients report previous experiences with ERP that have made them averse to the idea of conventional OCD treatment or skeptical that it can work for them.

In 2015, when I became acquainted with Internal Family Systems (IFS) therapy, it reminded me why I was drawn to psychotherapy in the first place. IFS is a collaborative and *experiential* form of therapy. With its emphasis on multiplicity and Self-leadership (described in Part I of this book), the IFS model is more attuned to the entire range of a client's present-moment experience than the psychodynamic approaches I originally studied and provides a framework for understanding and softening the dynamic struggles and interactions that go on within our psyches. It also resonated deeply with the principles of Buddhism and meditation I had been studying and practicing since the late 1980s. As I began to incorporate IFS into my practice, I started seeing the similarities between exposure therapy—especially as it is present in ACT—and the processes of the IFS model. For instance, both involve opening attention to whatever is arising in the present moment without being limited by avoidance or other protective strategies. And when I began to use exposure and IFS together, I started seeing remarkable results. With this combination of therapies, clients who were stuck or had plateaued began to get better.

This book is the result of nearly a decade of research, training, and experience, driven by my passion to find a more kind and comprehensive way for therapists to support the healing of individuals with OCD. The result is the therapeutic model I present here.

Introduction

A few short decades ago, obsessive-compulsive disorder (OCD) was misunderstood and egregiously underdiagnosed; its often seemingly bizarre symptoms were considered untreatable. Even today, the delay a person experiences between developing symptoms of OCD and receiving an accurate diagnosis and effective treatment is estimated to be between 11 and 17 years (García-Soriano et al., 2014). This has been due to a lack of awareness, stigma, and minimal access to effective providers trained in empirically validated methods for treating the disorder (Szymanski, 2012). Fortunately, all of that is improving. But still, only a small percentage of people with severe OCD are receiving evidence-based treatment with well-trained specialists. This problem has widespread ramifications: OCD is common, severe, and chronic. Throughout the world, the lifetime prevalence of OCD is 2–3% with 10% of people in psychiatric settings presenting with OCD symptoms (Brock & Hany, 2022). And, while the World Health Organization lists anxiety disorders, including OCD, as the "sixth largest contributor to non-fatal health loss globally" (WHO, 2017) and OCD as one of the top 10 leading causes of disability, *only* about 20% of people with OCD achieve remission over 40 years (Brock & Hany, 2022; Stein et al., 2019).

Given the prevalence, chronicity, and treatment challenges of OCD, a great deal of effort has recently gone into research aimed at establishing effective, evidence-based, frontline treatments. Specialized training in these methods is considered a prerequisite for providing OCD treatment. Most clinicians who specialize in treating OCD will tell you that unless you use an evidence-based approach—predominantly the traditional exposure and response prevention (ERP) model—you are not likely to see results. In fact, conventional talk therapy can actually do harm to clients with OCD by inadvertently reinforcing compulsive rumination and reassurance seeking. Unfortunately, specialists in evidence-based treatment of OCD are still relatively hard to find, so there is also a considerable gap in the sheer availability of treatment.

Many people with OCD respond well to exposure therapy. Roughly 60–80% of the clients who engage in ERP treatment experience at least a 35% reduction in their symptoms. Fewer, roughly 40%, experience more substantial relief, meaning about a 75% reduction in their symptoms (Abramowitz, 1998; Foa et al., 2012; McKay et al., 2015). That leaves a fairly large number of people who get part way there, but still struggle with ongoing limitations in their lives due to OCD symptoms.

Unfortunately, some clients do not respond as well to ERP, and others cannot or will not participate in it. In some cases, therapists may move too quickly and overwhelm a client, or slip into talk therapy rather than true exposure therapy. However, many well-trained and experienced OCD specialists find that some clients are unwilling to engage in exposure or they try it but hit roadblocks. In such instances, clinicians tend to pull back and address "treatment-interfering behaviors," or use motivational interviewing to enhance treatment readiness. However, all too often clients still hear recriminations: "You're not working hard enough." "Come back when you're ready." Even though ERP is considered the gold standard treatment for OCD, it's problematic to push someone through a treatment that they are not responding to, or to shame the client for lack of progress due to a "failure to comply."

Other factors, as well, can leave treatment at a standstill. Many clients with OCD also have co-occurring trauma or other diagnoses that make exposure therapy inadvisable or untenable. And recovery is further complicated by the fact that many people with OCD have, in addition, been traumatized by the very experience of having OCD, and ERP alone cannot address this spiral of trauma. Individuals with OCD often spent their childhoods thinking they were horrible people because of the gruesome, disturbing, or fearful thoughts or images that incessantly popped into their heads. As adults, these long-established internal, critical voices may sabotage treatment by reinforcing obsessions and compulsions and even creating an additional layer of depression or feelings of worthlessness, causing people to avoid therapy altogether because they don't feel they are worth saving. Further, the cascading real-life results of having OCD can create additional obstacles in both life and treatment—potentially resulting in loss of jobs and relationships, homelessness, hospitalizations, suicide attempts, and complete disability. And finally, for a variety of logistical reasons, treatment by OCD specialists trained in ERP is simply unavailable to many sufferers.

For all these reasons, the therapeutic community desperately needs a model of treatment that both maintains the angle and efficacy of exposure therapy and creates space to heal the psychological wounds that surround, bolster, and sometimes reinforce obsessive and compulsive symptoms. What if there was another way to help?

The approach to using Internal Family Systems (IFS) with OCD presented here evolved organically through my work with clients who often come to me with more than one concern and a list of diagnoses. I recognize that for those who are disabled by OCD, symptom relief may be the only thing that makes life worth living at all, and that of course comes first, but I value treatment that is attuned to the whole person. To address the complexities I was seeing, I found myself bringing an IFS approach into my ERP treatment. As I did, I began to see a strong overlap between the underlying principles of IFS and those of exposure therapy. As I continued to incorporate IFS into my work with clients with OCD, I realized that although some distinct features in OCD are critical to understand and appreciate, IFS could, with care, be used safely and effectively in the OCD population. In fact, integrating the approaches created a synergy that was having a powerful, life affirming impact.

I believe IFS therapy can provide the missing elements to help people who are falling though the treatment gap. The ways in which we can use and adjust IFS to accomplish this is the subject of the rest of the book. For now, I'll just say: IFS for OCD provides hope for people with OCD. It offers solutions for those who have not been helped or who have gotten somewhat better but are left with other pieces of themselves to pick up after treatment. Recovering from OCD no longer needs to leave clients feeling that they cannot trust themselves, that their minds are playing tricks on them, or that they need to accept that they "might or might not" be horrible people. Because IFS for OCD grounds its theory and practice in the IFS view of the internal world as a multiplicity within the context of an indestructible compassionate Self, it facilitates an inner sense of security and Self-trust that promotes healing in all domains of intrapsychic and interpersonal life. So the benefits for clients reach far beyond just reducing the symptoms of OCD.

And there are benefits for therapists as well. As I incorporated IFS into my work with OCD, I noticed not only the difference it was making for people who might otherwise not get help for their complex OCD but also the impact it had on the quality of my practice. As I became more Self-led as a therapist and began to notice, as I worked with clients, *who I was speaking to*—Self or a part—the whole process became more clear. When I apply the IFS lens, my clients get better and so does their OCD. In short, adding IFS makes ERP work better, and understanding ERP makes IFS work better with clients who have OCD. To that end, this book offers a summary of the theory and practice of IFS, an overview of OCD and evidence-based OCD treatment, and a theory and path to bring them together.

If you're an OCD specialist, I hope this book sparks your curiosity about IFS and offers an approach that will help you reach clients who need to experience treatment from a different angle. If you're an IFS clinician, I hope this book offers you enough insight into obsessional and compulsive protectors and related exiles, and the typical patterns that entrap them, to give you a greater sense of confidence in your work with OCD and an understanding of the ethical considerations regarding when to seek consultation, or refer out to a specialist or to a higher level of care. Above all, my intention is to offer options for those who need something more—not to undermine client participation in proven treatment methods for OCD.

What You'll Find in This Book

This book provides a theoretical approach to the treatment of OCD, developed through my work with clients and based on my clinical experiences. This book is divided into four parts.

To lay the foundation for an IFS-informed approach to OCD, Part I introduces IFS theory. Readers who are familiar with the IFS approach to therapy will find themselves on well-trodden ground, while those new to IFS will find an introduction to its basic perspectives and concepts in Chapter 1. Chapter 2 discusses the IFS process and methods.

Part II provides an essential overview of the mechanisms and processes of effective OCD treatment. Readers who already work with OCD will find themselves surefooted here, while those new to its standard treatment modalities will find information they must understand in order to treat the disorder effectively. Chapter 3 discusses OCD and its subtypes. Chapter 4 explains its traditional assessment and diagnosis. Chapter 5 discusses evidence-based treatment options for OCD, highlighting key clinical challenges and common errors that can sabotage its therapy.

Part III reconceptualizes OCD through the language of IFS theory, expanding the traditional view of the OCD cycle and introducing what I call the OC subsystem, setting it in the context of systems thinking and multiplicity of mind—the view that the human psyche comprises many interrelated parts rather than being a unitary structure. Chapter 6 presents the components of OCD—obsessions, compulsions, and core fears—in the language of IFS and offers an IFS view of the OC cycle. Chapter 7 expands on how the OC parts interact systemically to perpetuate the cycle. Chapter 8 provides a mapping of the mechanisms at work in IFS for OCD onto the effective processes and methods of evidence-based OCD treatment.

In Part IV, I explain *how* to use an IFS approach in the treatment of OCD, either alone or integrated with and augmenting traditional ERP protocols, providing a method for what I call Self-led ERP. Chapter 9 illustrates how OCD assessment may be done effectively within the IFS frame and the importance of this step as a foundation for successful treatment. Chapter 10 presents Stage One of Self-led ERP in which protective parts meet Self and give some permission establishing willingness and presence to move forward. Chapter 11 demonstrates Stage Two, an IFS version of exposure in which parts encounter previously exiled parts. In Chapter 12, Stage Three elucidates the further effort often needed with OC protectors to facilitate practice and engagement with the external system.

Melissa Mose
Calabasas, CA
July 2025

References

Abramowitz, J. S. (1998). Does cognitive-behavioral therapy cure obsessive-compulsive disorder? A meta-analytic evaluation of clinical significance. *Behavior Therapy*, 29(2), 339–355. https://doi.org/10.1016/S0005-7894(98)80012-9

Brock, H., & Hany, M. (2022). Obsessive-compulsive Disorder. In *StatPearls [Internet]*. StatPearls Publishing. https://www.ncbi.nlm.nih.gov/books/NBK553162/

Foa, E. B., Yadin, E., & Lichner, T. K. (2012). *Exposure and response (ritual) prevention for obsessive-compulsive disorder: Therapist guide* (2nd ed.). Oxford University Press.

García-Soriano, G., Rufer, M., Delsignore, A., & Weidt, S. (2014). Factors associated with non-treatment or delayed treatment seeking in OCD sufferers: A review of the literature. *Psychiatry Research*, 220(1–2), 1–10.

McKay, D., Sookman, D., Neziroglu, F., Wilhelm, S., Stein, D. J., Kyrios, M., Matthews, K., & Veale, D. (2015). Efficacy of cognitive-behavioral therapy for obsessive–compulsive disorder. *Psychiatry Research*, 227(1), 104–113. https://doi.org/10.1016/j.psychres.2015.02.004

Stein, D. J., Costa, D. L. C., Lochner, C., Miguel, E. C., Reddy, Y. C. J., Shavitt, R. G., Van Den Heuvel, O. A., & Simpson, H. B. (2019). Obsessive–compulsive disorder. *Nature Reviews Disease Primers*, 5(1), 52. https://doi.org/10.1038/s41572-019-0102-3

Szymanski, J. (2012). Using direct-consumer marketing strategies with obsessive-compulsive disorder in the nonprofit sector. *Behavior Therapy*, 43, 251–256.

World Health Organization. (2017). Depression and other common mental disorders: Global health estimates. World Health Organization.

Part I

Introduction to Internal Family Systems Therapy

Chapter 1

The Internal Family Systems Approach

In the universe around us, from solar systems to ecosystems to family systems, people recognize discrete parts interacting within a whole. Yet, until family therapist Richard Schwartz, PhD, developed the concept of Internal Family Systems (IFS) therapy, many psychotherapies failed to conceive of the internal world of the human psyche in such a way. Throughout his years as a family therapist working with clients with eating disorders, Schwartz paid close attention to the internal voices of his clients, noticing their similarity to dialogues in interpersonal relationships. Drawing on his experience as a family systems therapist, he developed an approach to individual therapy that mirrors the dynamics of interpersonal systems, demonstrating that our *intrapersonal* parts function in systems similar to the *external* family systems that we can more easily observe. The principles that govern systems of any type— mechanical, biological, or social—also function in the mind, and IFS therapy brings the dynamic complexity of systems thinking to the intrapsychic domain.

Balance between, and harmony among, the disparate parts of any system are key for its overall functioning. Just as families can have members with varying points of view and experiences, our own minds can hold multiple perspectives with simultaneously different or even contradictory thoughts and feelings. And just as family systems can have members who act out in ways that are disruptive to the whole, our own internal systems can be disturbed by intrapersonal conflicts. In both large and small systems, healing begins with valuing the individuals (in IFS, our *parts*) and learning why the extreme behavior is happening. The goal of IFS therapy is to bring the parts of a client's system back into balance with one another to create more stability and to foster harmony, understanding, and ultimately trust within.

This chapter introduces the basic perspective and concepts of IFS therapy.

The Self and Its Resources

The context of each person's internal system of parts is the essential *Self*, the IFS term for the clear and witnessing awareness or presence that is at the core of every human being. The Self is the inborn "seat of our consciousness," a universally innate and undamageable internal resource that is within us all (Schwartz & Sweezy, 2020, p. 45). Self is present in everyone, and it is always intact, whole, healthy, and undamaged, needing only to be uncovered in situations where it has been obscured. An apt analogy is that the Self is much like the sky—while it may be covered by clouds or smoke, it is still there when conditions clear up.

Schwartz founded IFS therapy on the belief that people have all of the internal resources that they need to achieve balance, resources he called the *8 C's*: compassion, curiosity, courage, creativity, connection, confidence, clarity, and calm (Schwartz, 2006). Where other therapeutic approaches may conceptualize these internal resources as skills to be developed or states to be achieved, Schwartz insisted that they need only to be uncovered if they are buried; he found compassion, for example, to be already present and undamaged in even the most apparently hardened clients (Goulding & Schwartz, 2002, p. 82).

The primary goal of IFS therapy is to free up a client's internal resources, to restore vitality to the whole internal system, and to re-establish the Self as the leader and primary healing capacity of the person.

A Multiplicity of Mind

As Schwartz observed the internal dialogues of his clients, he noticed that they would regularly use the phrase "part of me" to refer to a state of mind that they experienced as recurring with some regularity. For example, they would express internal conflicts by saying "Part of me knows I should get some exercise, but another part of me would rather just sit on the couch and watch TV" or "Part of me is really angry at so and so, but I know they didn't mean to be hurtful." These explanations of inner disputes happened so often that Schwartz came to understand them not as metaphors, but as accurate descriptions of his clients' internal realities. What they called their "parts" acted much like independent people with their own motives, beliefs, goals, and agendas, displaying patterns of relating to the world that ranged from balanced and effective to extreme, polarized, and dysfunctional. These multiple parts had internal relationships with one another that functioned very much like the relationships he had seen in family systems: Just as with members of a family, some parts seemed to be on the same page, some misunderstood each other, and some were in frank opposition.

Imagine a common situation involving interactions among your own internal parts. At a friend's house, you're offered a slice of cake. Multiple thoughts run through your mind:

That looks delicious, and I deserve a treat, a part of you thinks with delight.
But I really shouldn't eat all that sugar, another part of you cautions.
Still, I don't want to be rude, a third part rationalizes.
Maybe just one or two bites, a fourth part proposes.

As amazing as it is to recognize all the voices crowding in to comment on this one simple choice, it's typical for all of us to constantly experience similar internal conversations among the "parts of me."

Formally positing that "the human mind is naturally divided into parts" (Goulding & Schwartz, 2002, p. 9), Schwartz began to use *parts* as a technical term. He also noticed that in contrast to the behaviors that clients described as parts of their personalities, they often described an internal sense of presence that they referred to as the "real me"—the *Self*. Self is the compassionate context within which parts, and the complex relationships among them, play out. Uniting the concepts of parts and Self in the phrase *multiplicity of mind* to describe the structure and functioning of human awareness with its many internal voices, points of view, moods, and behavioral tendencies, Schwartz articulated a system of therapy that is both nuanced and pragmatic, potentially useful in treating many psychological issues or diagnoses.

Initially, it's helpful to think of the parts of our personalities as states of mind or patterns of behavior that recur often enough to become familiar and easily recognizable. We have different moods, tendencies, and traits that we experience as familiar thoughts, feelings, sensations, images, or urges. Each of our parts has a particular concern and originates from an intention to help us. When our parts are integrated and balanced under the leadership of the Self, their roles and qualities contribute positively to our overall functioning and work harmoniously toward a common goal. However, when burdened, out of balance, and extreme, their limited perspectives cause them to work at cross purposes with one another.

In the example above, imagine that you accept the slice of cake you're offered. You take that first bite, savoring its flavor, and then another. Before you know it, you've had far more than the two bites you decided to eat. Now a new set of parts chime in:

I'm an undisciplined slob, a part of you cries in disgust.
How am I ever going to accomplish anything if I can't set a simple intention and stick to it? another part worries.
Now I'm miserable, a third part moans.
And it serves me right, a fourth part pronounces.

The voices that first deliberated your actions are joined by a crowd of voices reacting to their results—and not liking the results. And these parts are only too willing to blame and shame you if that's what they believe it will take to protect you.

When parts take over, they assume temporary leadership of the system and—given their partial perspectives—they often create internal conflict; if the patterns persist, intensify, and become destructive, they eventually present to the therapist as symptoms of a psychological disorder. But even under such circumstances, it's a tenet of IFS therapy that there are "no bad parts" (Schwartz, 2021). All parts of an internal system deserve to be respected, listened to, and allowed to share their understanding of the whole person. That's because even our perceived inner enemies—parts that act out in ways that harm us (eating or drinking to excess, for example)—originally developed as solutions to counter something else causing an imbalance. The goal of IFS therapy is to help those parts find a path to beneficial ways of operating—not to ignore them, suppress them, or otherwise try to control or change them.

Where another approach to therapy might try to eradicate "bad" behaviors, IFS therapy succeeds by approaching the behaviors with curiosity to learn what motivates them. Anyone who has tried to change a longstanding pattern (by dieting, for instance) has likely noticed that strategies of control work only for a period of time, then a rebound process takes over and undoes progress. Even though some parts may want to change, other parts will have different ideas about what's best. By valuing the input of all members of a person's internal system, an IFS therapist establishes a non-pathologizing working environment in which to help clients identify impediments to healthy functioning.

Self-Leadership

The guiding principle of IFS theory is that a system in harmony with itself is *Self-led*. With Self in the leadership role, the internal qualities of the 8 C's provide wellbeing, even in hard times, as a person's Self exudes a sense of calm. Instead of identifying with one state of mind, a Self-led person is conscious of having (not *being*) thoughts, feelings, and urges, and can witness them as they ebb and flow, releasing a wellspring of *Self-energy*. This larger perspective frees Self to consider the points of view of all the various parts when making decisions and mediating among their sometimes competing needs for the good of the system as a whole.

With Self in charge, people live authentically, with awareness of their parts in harmonious participation with one another. Often, however, Self is crowded out; to a greater or lesser degree, Self is overshadowed by a singular state of mind, and a person identifies with only one or a few perspectives—forgetting, denying, or rejecting others. When the desires and agendas of parts take over, Self is no longer in the driver's seat. Schwartz calls this state being *blended* with one or more parts, and he demonstrated that people, when blended, lose the ability to make clear, conscious choices. We find ourselves behaving repeatedly in ways we wish we hadn't or failing to accomplish what we set out to do. "I don't know why I do that," we say. "I don't know why that always happens."

When we are blended with the thoughts, feelings, and activities of our parts, we allow them to cloud our awareness and limit access to curiosity and other positive qualities of Self. When we are *moderately* blended with a part, we are influenced by its perspective and act according to its tendencies and traits. This limits our contact with reality and can leave us feeling lost and disconnected, unable to know with any true clarity how we feel, what we want, and how to choose. When we are *highly* blended, we actually see ourselves, others, and the world through the eyes of the over-active part. With a part in the driver's seat, we become stuck on one track, making decisions that fail to make room for all of our needs.

Unblending from Parts

When the desires and agendas of one or more parts take over consistently, Self may not even be in the passenger's seat, but quiet or hidden in the back of the bus. And so, the first phase of IFS therapy is primarily concerned with *unblending*: The process of noticing parts and helping them become differentiated from Self and one another. The more willing parts are to unblend, the more we can understand our internal conflicts and build internal relationships that are more balanced, productive, and harmonious, with the Self in the lead. In helping clients to develop this ability, IFS therapists offer clients the tools to help their extreme parts return to their original, preferred roles, allowing the whole nervous system to settle (Schwartz & Sweezy, 2020). In the moment that a part is acknowledged, Self is activated, a shift occurs, and a relationship is regained. Developing this perspective—uncomfortable at first—begins the process of fostering internal relationships that are trusting and secure, an ongoing goal of IFS.

In order to restore Self to its leadership role, IFS therapists help clients understand their parts' multifaceted natures, motivations, and messages. The first step in unblending is to help clients develop the ability to detect and differentiate from parts, simply by acknowledging them. (Chapter 2 delves into these techniques.) The more effectively clients can notice, describe, and observe their parts, the more readily those parts will cooperate in the process of unblending to make space for Self.

Schwartz found that the simple act of helping clients to externalize and name their parts fostered curiosity, perspective, and a clearer way to relate to them. Certain types of parts—critics and avoidant parts for instance—are common and appear to some degree in nearly everyone. Other typical parts include perfectionistic or compliant parts that attempt to protect a person from feeling inadequate; zoned-out parts that spend too much time scrolling; and impulsive parts that overspend or use substances to find relief from an overwhelmed or pressured system. Helping clients identify their parts and listen to them facilitates the unblending process. The idea is to help clients move out of speaking *from the part* ("I'm so angry!") to speaking *for the part* ("a part of me is angry"). This reframing usually creates a palpable and noticeable shift in the client's sense of control.

Let's identify some parts that may have interacted in the above scenario.

The dessert looks appealing, and a soothing part of you wants to reward you with cake.
A controlling or inhibiting health-conscious part of you warns of negative impact.
A polite, people-pleasing part joins the side of the one who wants cake.
A Self-like negotiator proposes a compromise.

Soon, a whole new set of your parts may have joined the fray.

A harsh inner critic calls you names because you lost control.
A worried part catastrophizes about the future and generalizes the lack of control to the rest of your life endeavors.
A punishing part adds blame and shame to the discomfort of being full.

In time, after getting comfortable with the process of identifying and externalizing parts, clients who are able to see recurring patterns in their own behavior may take the lead and create proper names that reflect the specific life experiences of their parts: For example, a client may spontaneously offer that the "angry part of me" is not just angry; instead, it's a "Fireball"—and renaming the part as "Fireball" may make room for the client to recognize that the part has additional, perhaps more valuable, jobs than anger. The parts clients name may be of any age, any gender; they may be adopted from pop culture or from their personal lives. Fascinatingly, the names clients assign to their parts often evolve over the course of therapy as they achieve greater clarity and appreciation for them.

Returning to our not-so-simple example:

I deserve a treat. (That's your Cookie Monster—om nom nom!)
But I really shouldn't eat all that sugar. (Health Nut, always there and always so superior.)
Still, I don't want to be rude. (Miss Manners, on the job.)

Maybe just one or two bites. (Self talking? No: Actually your Rationalizer making excuses while pretending to be objective.)
I'm an undisciplined slob. (Totally your Mean Girl.)
How am I ever going to accomplish anything if I can't set a simple intention and stick to it? (Ugh. End-of-the-World guy.)
Now I'm miserable. (Hi, Eeyore.)
And it serves me right. (Sigh. That's Mr. Know-It-All.)

By personifying your parts, you begin to understand their preoccupations and concerns, which helps you view them with compassion.

Alliances and Polarizations

When the Self is sufficiently accessible, all of the parts of a person's psyche are willingly encountered, welcomed, and expressed—including parts that represent uncomfortable feelings and beliefs. This state of healthy balance supports a fluidity that allows people to move in and out of various states of mind or parts, with relative freedom, bringing our individual capacities to bear when relevant and allowing them to recede when not needed. With Self in the lead, we are clear-headed, present, mindful, aware of our feelings, and able to manage the requirements of our daily lives. When our minds are unbalanced and chaotic, however—when parts usurp leadership and occlude Self—individual parts (or teams of them) compete for dominance in a struggle for supremacy.

Parts with aligned interests and compatible methods begin to pursue their own ends, supporting one another in a variety of ways ranging from simple validation to teaming up and lending resources. A critical part may team up with a perfectionist, for instance, forming an internal *alliance* that endeavors to prevent mistakes and improve inadequacies. As one of my clients explained, her Food-Restricting part and her Straight-A's part worked closely with her critical part, whom she called Mean Girl, to make sure that she would have a "successful future."

Alternately, parts of us can become *polarized*, opposing either the values or the methods of the others, and fighting to undo the work of another part or team of parts. A polarization occurs when parts work against one another—each protector undoing the other's work, becoming more extreme in order to counteract or counterbalance the work of the other, who also becomes more extreme. Each part is convinced that if the other has its way—even just a little bit—it would do something destructive, resulting in disaster. For instance, a reactive, disinhibitory firefighter may eat to counteract the overly restrictive, inhibitory work of a manager striving for control over body weight. Neither realizes that the other has the same big-picture goal and is just going about reaching it in a different way. In the service of what might seem to be a common goal, the two parts compete, causing confusing and contradictory behavior in the person they're trying to protect—a classic case of internal polarization.

As another client struggles with a health decision, I watch her vacillate between one part that wants to do the right thing for long-term health and another part that wants a quick fix by taking a medication that's harder on the body but works faster. Where is Self in that struggle? Parts, with their partial perspectives, can battle for dominance in a system, working effectively and relentlessly to undo the work of other parts, who are similarly determined to have their way. When locked into these opposing positions, polarized parts make it feel impossible to make a choice or take any action, immobilizing the person and clouding their sense of Self.

Vulnerable Parts and Protective Parts

In a Self-led system, *vulnerable parts* are cherished and kept safe and secure by mild-mannered *protective parts*—those who balance drive and moderation, reasonable caution and a willingness to try new things, functioning as adults watching over beloved children. These protective parts represent our capacities, gifts, skills, and traits, and they are a rich source of information about the delicate balance of parts within a personality. For instance, someone who is gifted with a great sense of humor and finds it easy to make others laugh may lean on a humorous part to balance out a more vulnerable shy part that it protects.

When a mind is out of balance, however, it experiences the openness of vulnerable parts as threats to the system. For instance, if the shy part becomes more extreme and socially anxious, it stirs up even more distress and possibly immobilization. As these parts accumulate pain, the formerly benign efforts of protectors can become extreme, imposing behavioral constraints and limiting a person's freedom to act and react with spontaneity and flexibility. That humorous part might become a Class Clown or Practical Jokester who, by becoming so out of touch with its impact on others, makes enemies instead of friends.

Burdens and Exiles

As a way of coping with psychic pain in the form of toxic beliefs, intolerable memories, discomfort, confusion, and extreme fear—pain that Schwartz called *burdens*—protective parts seek to quiet the vulnerable parts, much as exasperated adults might scold or shush children when they're acting out. Their motive may be to protect the vulnerable parts from drawing negative attention; they may, instead, be blaming the vulnerable parts for causing their own discomfort. In either case, protectors may become harsh and even cruel in the name of doing their jobs if the feelings carried by vulnerable parts are too hurtful or frightening to be held in the forefront of awareness. One part may get loud and use name calling and criticism as a method of motivation; another part, feeling attacked, may seek relief through self-harm rather than an innocuous method such as watching TV.

By banishing a person's vulnerable parts, protective parts turn them into *exiles*, parts that surface in therapy feeling unloved, abandoned, scared of other people, or confused by others' behavior. Some exiles, carrying memories of being hurt, show up as sensations of heaviness or darkness, or as physical symptoms such as stomach pain or shakiness. All exiles carry the burdens—the painful thoughts, feelings, and sensations—saddled on them by the protective parts of the system. In their single-minded attempts to keep the person safe (*untriggered*), the protectors lose touch with the impact they have on the person they are intending to protect. The qualities of Self are less available, which leads to further internal instability and unpredictability and invites even more intense activity to keep the exiled parts out of awareness.

The vulnerable parts, however, don't want to be alone. Objecting to their forced exile, they begin to amplify their voices, becoming an ever-greater threat that floods the person with fear and pain. In extreme cases, exiles may succeed in taking over, causing a person to feel chronically overwhelmed by negative thoughts and feelings, creating observable symptoms.

Managers and Firefighters

Although the psyche of each individual contains highly personal internal parts, each with its own specific interests and concerns, those parts also take on *roles* common to internal systems in general. Some protective parts take on *proactive* responsibilities; they structure, control, plan, and carry out the activities of daily life. Schwartz called this type of role a *manager*. Other parts take on more *reactive* responsibilities, dealing with the consequences of our actions, especially when perceiving problems or threats. Schwartz called this type of role a *firefighter*. Together the parts that inhabit these roles provide safety and security for the system as a whole.

Proactive Managers

Managers are the parts of ourselves that we rely on to navigate life. When we say, "I have to check my calendar" or "I can't stand being late," we're talking from the parts of us that work as managers. Our managers set the alarm for the morning, plan the day, and play nicely with others at work or school. They work to maintain control of the environment, prevent mistakes, and keep us on track so that we don't feel bad or risk harm. They push us to achieve and perform, and they hide our imperfections. Much of the time, we intentionally count on our manager parts to accomplish the things we intend to do and help us be the way we intend to be.

Although our managers can be quite helpful when balanced and working in harmony with other parts, they can also become driven and extreme when they feel that a person's survival depends on them doing what they do. Some examples of extreme managers are parts that exhibit perfectionistic, vigilant, critical, obsessive, or people-pleasing behaviors. In seeking to prevent actual danger, fear, pain, or other vulnerability, they can inadvertently *cause* problems as they double down on their efforts to "manage" feelings that have not been addressed.

Because managers have a rationale for their work—to prevent vulnerable parts from surfacing with all their feelings—they will become louder and more demanding if they feel their moderate efforts are not enough. They always have good intentions, but because they are only parts of us, and therefore have limited vision, they don't have the clarity and perspective of Self. They may not understand that it's the role of Self to preside and that it's all right for them to relax back into their preferred, subordinate roles.

Reactive Firefighters

Firefighters are the parts of us that take action when danger arises internally. When we say, "I need a drink!" or "That's it, I'm through with this!" we're talking from the parts of us that work as firefighters. No matter how hard our managers work to keep things in order and functioning, there are times when we feel the pain of embarrassment, failure, loss, or frustration. Because we generally can't just give into those feelings and let them take over—we have to continue to do our jobs or appear stable to those around us—we need some mechanism to help us set these feelings aside so we can carry on. That's the role of firefighters, who, like managers, can be mild and helpful but can also become extreme and more reactive over time.

From uncomfortable and inconvenient to seemingly intolerable, painful feelings exist on a continuum and require different levels of urgency and extremity for relief. For milder pain, distraction and self-soothing (shopping, flirting, playing video games) may suffice as short-term solutions to shift focus and "fix" the feelings. In more extreme cases, self-destructive behaviors such as self-harm, binge eating, drug or alcohol abuse, and dissociation can emerge as attempts to neutralize the pain and terror of trauma. These behaviors inevitably create additional problems down the line.

Like all our parts, firefighters have a range of emotions from mild to extreme. Regardless of the consequences, and depending on the level of pain, firefighters use whatever means they have to extinguish the flames of a difficult experience, and they don't mind or notice if they do damage in the process. Their methods are not designed to be careful and subtle, but to have a large and immediate impact: relief.

Although it's obvious how damaging certain firefighter behaviors can become—spending a person into debt, eating into an unhealthy state, etc.—even seemingly innocuous behaviors such as making sure a door is locked can get out of control and create disastrous consequences in a person's life, taking up many hours of a person's day.

As with managers, all firefighters—even extreme firefighters—have good intentions, but they, too, are only parts of us with limited vision. It's not their goal to take over or take on extreme roles; instead, they are motivated by fears or concerns about what might happen if they don't do their jobs. IFS therapy helps them return to their preferred roles.

The Goals of IFS Therapy

The overarching goal of IFS therapy is to help clients re-establish Self as the primary leader of their internal systems, restoring trust in Self. More than acquiring new skills, people need to be released from constraints imposed upon them by the negative self-referential beliefs and the strong feelings of fear and terror that lead to behaviors that distort their lives and, in therapy, are noted as symptoms. Therefore, as Schwartz and Sweezy note (2020, p. 106), the practice of IFS therapy has three primary experiential goals:

> (1) [l]iberating parts from extreme roles so they can move on to preferred, valued roles; (2) restoring the trust of parts in the leadership of the Self; [and] (3) re-harmonizing the system of parts such that they get to know each other and form productive collaborations.

The underlying problem that IFS therapy addresses is the unbalanced and chaotic mind that results when Self is not available to lead. Understanding that the human psyche is composed of parts and that each person is a psychic multiplicity, IFS therapy guides people to turn their focus inward and pay attention to the dynamics between and among their individual parts, acknowledging their disparate motivations and agendas while seeking to understand their constructive intentions (Sweezy, 2023).

References

Goulding, R. A., & Schwartz, R. C. (2002). *The mosaic mind: Empowering the tormented selves of child abuse survivors*. Trailheads.

Schwartz, R. C. (2006). *Internal family systems therapy*. Recording for the Blind & Dyslexic.

Schwartz, R. C. (2021). *No bad parts: Healing trauma & restoring wholeness with the internal family systems model*. Sounds True.

Schwartz, R. C., & Sweezy, M. (2020). *Internal family systems therapy* (2nd ed.). The Guilford Press.

Sweezy, M. (2023). *Internal family systems therapy for shame and guilt*. The Guilford Press.

Chapter 2

The Process and Methods of IFS Therapy

Internal Family Systems (IFS) therapy takes place in two non-linear (and often interwoven) phases: (1) earning the willingness of protectors to unblend and (2) attending to the needs of exiles. In the first phase, the IFS therapist helps protective parts trust that they can safely unblend, so clients can experience their internal systems as differentiated—and consciously perceive the noncontrolling attitude of Self and the reality that they *have* parts rather than that they *are* parts. In the second phase, the IFS therapist guides clients to encounter and form positive relationships between the Self and the exiled parts, helping these more vulnerable parts feel understood and accepted so they can let go of their burdens. Once freed from these negative beliefs, exiles are able to rejoin the whole system, offering their assets and capacities in an integrated and harmonious way (Schwartz & Sweezy, 2020). In practice, these two phases—unblending and healing—are not distinct, tending to flow back and forth, but it is helpful to separate them for purposes of instruction.

This chapter introduces the process and methods of IFS therapy. It begins with a discussion of the qualities of the IFS therapist and then continues by describing the basics steps in each of the two phases of IFS. This chapter concludes with a discussion of methods IFS therapists often use to facilitate unblending and unburdening.

The Qualities of the IFS Therapist

IFS therapy differs from some other therapeutic approaches in its foundational focus on the Self of the *therapist*. As IFS therapists, our ongoing task is to be Self-led, to cultivate Self-energy, and to develop and maintain our own conscious, healthy *Self-to-part* relationships—a powerful commitment that ensures a truly compassionate environment for our clients.

IFS therapists practice being aware of our own parts, as they inevitably show up in the therapeutic process with their own concerns, opinions, and personalities. Therapy is an intense set of encounters, and some of our parts are likely to get activated during interactions with our clients. For example, it's not uncommon for therapists to have parts that are tired or aren't looking forward to a certain session or parts that resonate with what the client is reporting. When that happens, IFS therapists notice our activated parts and help them unblend, when appropriate, sometimes out loud and in real time. In this way, we model the process of *witnessing* and unblending, and we demonstrate results that our clients can see and feel. We might say, "I have a part that is really relating to you right now, and I imagine that your experience is different than mine, so could you say more about how that was for you?" This kind of description and inquiry helps both our own parts feel acknowledged and the client's parts feel seen as unique, yet connected.

IFS therapists are also aware of our *therapist parts* with their own agendas about how a given therapeutic intervention is progressing. For example, when a client has firefighters that are extreme, such as suicidal or self-harming parts, our own therapist parts may want to jump in with safety plans, goals for emotion regulation, or a manualized technique. True, our therapeutic agendas are developed from our training as well as our experience with other clients, and they offer valuable context for the therapeutic encounter. Also true: While no two people are the same, common patterns operate in the human psyche, and we can harness our understanding of those dynamics to fuel our confidence and our compassion. Internally acknowledging that we have these tools and accessing the qualities of Self, we can unblend from that skillful therapist part and maintain our full attention on the client so that we are open and can listen to all that the client's system actually needs in the moment.

To help our clients, IFS therapists must be both firm and resolute, yet also curious and open. In this way, we demonstrate having the courage to sit in "not knowing" while remaining calm and clear in that uncertainty. This state of curiosity, when we are able to hold it during our work, is the most therapeutic element in IFS. It allows us to keep from diving into "figuring out," "calming down," or "reassuring and soothing"—all fixes that our clients may think they want from us, but that might be counterproductive. The 5 P's are qualities that Schwartz emphasized as particularly valuable for IFS therapists to embody, and which many therapists naturally embody when they are Self-led: presence, patience, persistence, perspective, and playfulness (Schwartz & Sweezy, 2020). Because IFS therapy is attuned to and responsive to the moment-to-moment changes in the client's system, keeping these qualities in mind facilitates the discernment needed to be optimally attuned and respectful while also facilitating growth in the ways most needed and desired by the client.

Knowing Our Own Internal Systems

For therapists as well as for our clients, our individual parts, like distinct internal family members, represent our many capacities and embody our personality traits. They also engage in dynamic relationships that grow, change, and influence each other. It's natural that many, if not most, of our parts are aligned and contribute their strengths to valued activities and life goals. It's also natural for our parts to disagree, hold different perspectives, and sometimes work in opposite directions to counterbalance one another.

In order to be the trustworthy presence our clients need to guide their own inner work, IFS therapists begin by attending to our own internal systems and gauging our own level of Self-energy. We do this by taking ourselves through unblending, the first stage of IFS therapy, on our own, doing our own internal check-in, ideally before we start each session. This check-in might consist simply of asking ourselves questions such as, *What feelings do I notice? What thoughts? How much internal space do I have?* Or it may involve taking ourselves through the 6 F's described below.

We also check in with ourselves as the session progresses. As therapy unfolds, we may find that we have concerns about the work, agendas for the client, or reactions to the information or feelings that the client reveals. We may recognize that we have parts holding negative feelings or sensations—protectors leaping into action or exiles in distress or pain that respond to our clients' pain. By noticing our parts with gratitude, hearing their wisdom, and gently asking them to step back, we refresh our natural ability to be present without being crowded by thoughts and feelings so we can better help our clients experience their own parts in their individual ways. While it takes practice to be able to flow through the check-in process with ease, by doing so we are able to stay attuned to Self in a way that demonstrates to our clients our mutual humanity and facilitates their process of learning to do the same.

The Process of IFS Therapy

The process of IFS therapy differs fundamentally from standard therapy approaches, including both psychodynamic talk therapy and cognitive behavioral therapy. Using a family systems model, it applies that understanding of dynamics and relationships to the internal world of the client. In order to accomplish this goal, IFS is not analytical or programmatic. The protocol is experiential, and it often involves inviting clients to close their eyes, as one would do in a guided meditation process. In an IFS session, however, the therapist does not follow a predetermined script, instead maintaining a loose structure that allows the client's Self to make connections with parts and to choose which paths to follow. It does, however, proceed in two phases. The beginning phase involves building trust with protectors to secure their willingness to unblend. The second phase turns attention toward the needs of the exiled parts.

Building Trust with Protectors: Unblending and Befriending

The first phase of IFS therapy is primarily focused on helping the client to first notice protectors, and then help protectors become willing to unblend. This process encourages and facilitates the development of a trusting relationship with the Self of the client (and the therapist) in which the protector parts feel understood, acknowledged, and even appreciated. With unblending and *befriending*, in which we signal our differentiated acknowledgment and acceptance, the kind attention of Self becomes increasingly pervasive.

In this first phase, we begin by seeking answers to two related questions. The first involves learning what parts are holding the client's symptoms. Symptoms can serve two purposes: They can arise—either proactively or reactively—from protectors' attempts to prevent a person from experiencing uncomfortable feelings, and/or they can result from the periodic, overwhelming attempts of exiles clamoring to be acknowledged and attended to. The IFS therapist's first assessment is to learn whether the client's symptomatic parts are protectors, exiles, or both.

The second question is how much access the client has to Self in the present moment; the answer determines how we work with the client in the beginning phases of therapy. When clients exhibit a calm demeanor and open-minded curiosity toward their parts, it suggests they have access to Self. The more they use words that suggest any of the 8 C's—compassion, curiosity, courage, creativity, connection, confidence, clarity, and calm—the more that clients are likely to be Self-led. Observing their demeanor offers clues as well. When Self-led, people speak more slowly, quietly, and thoughtfully. Their postures are relaxed, and their ability to connect with the therapist is notable.

Differentiating between Protector Parts and the Self

Systems seek equilibrium. In a balanced, Self-led system, parts recognize and trust the presence of Self. They exert their effort when called upon and settle down when appropriate. But because our internal parts function as "separate centers of motivation" (Sweezy, 2023), they have different perspectives, each with its own validity, and thus different strategies for their behavior. IFS therapy seeks to facilitate a shift of consciousness that allows people to see and understand all their parts more clearly, track the parts' reactions to each other, and appreciate all of them as related to, but not the same as, Self. This shift promotes Self-energy, which has a gentle quality, a kindness about it, that brings inclusive, non-controlling attention—and the distance, perspective, and clarity that comes with it—to all sides.

Going Inside

A person's ability to pause and ponder about a part demonstrates some distance from it. IFS therapists begin therapy through a process we call *going inside*, a phrase for directing attention to internal experiences in the mind and body. We ask our clients to turn their attention inward—often by closing their eyes, if they find that comfortable—focusing on what is being experienced in the moment, including thoughts, feelings, sensations, or imagery. Some therapists close their eyes as well; either way, our initial task is primarily to help clients identify their parts as they arise by reflecting what they say back to them in parts language.[1] For instance, we might say something like the following:

> Close your eyes if you're comfortable or just lower them in a soft gaze. Turn your attention inside and notice what you're experiencing in your mind and body. Pay attention to whatever is arising. Many parts communicate through words or show us images; some show up as feelings, sensations, or urges. See if a part or parts of you would like your attention right now.
>
> If you sense a part that wants your attention, notice how you became aware of it. Is it making itself known as a voice or using your body, through a visual, a memory, a feeling, or a sense impression? If it feels OK, let the part know you recognize it and invite the part to share more of itself with you.

The process of identifying parts is different for everyone. Some people have a multisensory experience of their parts, meaning that they see them in their mind's eye, and hear their voices as distinct from their own. Or they may simply feel their parts as pressure, buzzing, or a sense of calm. There's no right or wrong way to experience parts when a person goes inside. What matters is that we help our clients notice and engage with their own experiences in whatever way works for them so that we can help them acknowledge and befriend the part, then—if the part is a protective part—ask it for permission to access and help the vulnerable part or parts that it's protecting.

When our clients' protective parts feel acknowledged and trusting, they become willing to unblend and allow access to the healing presence of their Self-energy. And when we are clear and Self-led in our roles as therapists, we are able to confidently acknowledge that even parts that behave dangerously or destructively have good intentions. We understand that these parts would gladly be moderate if they felt they could, that is, if they knew that there was a Self who could lead with confidence. We help them get to this place by first acknowledging them and asking them why they do what they do. Parts usually find this attention disarming and reassuring and soften a bit as a result of our sincere curiosity.

We engage in the process of parts detection throughout therapy, but in this first phase of treatment, we do so to discover which part or parts seem most urgently related to the client's symptoms. If clients are unaware of parts they are blended with, and can't find one that wants attention, we speak directly with parts that are obvious, without drawing attention to the fact that that's what we're doing. However, often parts do present themselves for work. Because it's the nature of exiled parts to be hidden, the parts that initially surface are likely to be protective parts—managers or firefighters—that engage in methodical or impulsive behaviors to keep the exiles hidden. We call a protective part that has presented itself for work the *target part*.

If a client has successfully made contact with a target part, we have some choices that depend upon the client's experiences with the protective part. Is the client able to experience Self as separate from the part, even momentarily? We gauge the level of this ability by noticing whether or not the client can speak *for* a part or is always identified with it, and if the client can be curious about or interested in the part or hates it and wants to be rid of it. If the client is unable to connect to Self, we step in with our own Self-energy to support the dialogue with the target part. Our modeling of compassionate attunement will eventually help clients find those qualities in themselves as they deepen their knowledge of their own systems.

Some protective parts are reluctant to relinquish their territory. Although people are commonly able to acknowledge their different parts and conflicting desires ("part of me wants *this*, but part of me wants *that*"), clients can become so blended with a single part, completely identifying with that singular perspective, that they lose contact with their sense of Self and any awareness of other parts with thoughts and feelings. IFS values the compassionate connection with parts that can arise only with a little distance from them. The more effectively clients can step back, notice, describe, and observe their parts, the more their parts feel seen and acknowledged and the more readily they will be willing to cooperate with the request to make space for Self.

Unblending involves stepping back from the part or asking it to step back and give more space. Because unblending from protective parts is the key to accessing Self, IFS therapists aim to facilitate it as early as possible in therapy. Clinically, we know that a client's parts are blended when the client is not experiencing at least one of the 8 C's that represent qualities of Self. In that case, we listen for parts that may have agendas and help those parts unblend. To help parts unblend, we engage in a step-by-step process called the *6 F's*: Find, Focus On, Flesh Out, Feel Toward, BeFriend, and Identify Fears.

Step 1: Find

By sitting with a client during the process of going inside, we discover the thoughts, feelings, sensations, or images that the client is experiencing in the present moment. These clues to the client's inner states are called *trailheads*—illuminating avenues of exploration that often lead us to parts, drives, needs, and motivations. Often we discover these trailheads by asking how a part is showing up in or around the body. Some people feel the part; others see or hear it. We follow clients' experience and help them notice more of it.

Step 2: Focus On

Having identified the few or the many parts that present themselves, we guide the client to notice which one needs immediate attention. This will be the initial target part. If you are unsure whether the part is a protector or an exile, ask if it has a job or if it protects anyone. If it says no, it's an exile. In IFS therapy, we always trust the clients' parts to know who they are and what they do. If the part you'd identified as your initial target part is an exile, ask it to wait for attention, letting it know that you will return when you can. If the part tells you that it protects a part or does something else important—or if you get no answer—then it's a protector.

Step 3: Flesh Out

Next, we guide clients to begin to differentiate parts from Self by asking them to notice details about the target part. Does it speak with a certain type of voice? Is it close or far? If they see it, what does it look like? Is it colorful? Textured? Big or small? Do they notice any particular qualities such as aggression or evasiveness? If they sense the part, how do they know it's there?

Step 4: Feel Toward

Once clients have begun to focus more intently on a part, we ask them how they feel *toward* the part (given what they may be discovering about it). This question allows us to check how much Self-energy is available to the client. Usually, a part has an opinion about what is being explored. It may be a part that wants to figure out what it means or how it got there, or it may respond with hostility. The answer to "How do you feel toward this part?" will suggest the extent to which clients are in touch with Self, or whether they are seeing a given part through the eyes of another part.

If they are accessing Self, they will most likely respond with some language that is reminiscent of the 8 C's. For instance, they may express compassion by saying, "I feel for it," or acceptance and connection by saying, "I get it." Responses such as these, which convey a sense of calm, or clarity, indicate access to Self. On the other hand, responses such as "It scares me," "I hate it," or "I am so frustrated with it" indicate the presence of another part reacting to the target part. Acknowledge any other parts that show up with reactions that don't align with the 8 C's and help them to feel heard, so they'll relax and step back. If they will, we check again to see how the client is feeling toward the target part. If any part won't, then it becomes the new target part, and we begin anew. We do not move on to the last two of the 6 F's until a person is somewhat Self-led and can feel toward the parts from a position of genuine curiosity. We return to Step 4 periodically whenever a part with an agenda is sitting in the driver's seat.

Step 5: BeFriend

When the client feels curiosity, kindness, or compassion toward the target part, we are in the presence of Self and can guide them to ask the part some questions. Try to allow your own curiosity to suggest the questions; some standard ones to consider are: How long have you been a part of this person? Do you have a message? Are you trying to say something? What do you do for [the client]? Who or what parts do you have conflicts or disagreements with, and who or what parts do you like or align with? Do you like your job? Do you work too hard? If the part has issues with or is afraid of another protector, offer to help with that conflict.

Step 6: Identify Fears

When the client is sufficiently differentiated from the target part, guide the client to inquire into the job the part does for the system and ask the part what it thinks might happen if it stopped. The goal of this step is to identify the part of the client that the target part protects. If it names a vulnerable part (an exile), we move directly into the next phase of therapy, offering to help that exile heal. This final step of the 6 F's helps foster trust between Self and parts because it encourages the target part to explain its reality, how it came to take on its role, and what keeps it hard at work whether its behavior is wanted or unwanted.

As this first portion of IFS therapy resolves for now, we have earned the willingness of the relevant protectors. Once they feel and trust the inviting qualities of Self they can give their permission to turn toward the exile. As other protective parts come up or the original target parts become concerned, we will return to the 6 F's and facilitate unblending and befriending again. This happens throughout therapy.

Attending to the Needs of Exiles: The Healing Steps

The second phase of IFS therapy consists of an impactful method we call the *healing steps*—a process that helps clients shift the dynamics of their internal systems and facilitate their ability to develop secure Self-to-part relationships. This process works primarily with exiled parts once the protective system has relaxed enough to allow the Self to be truly available. Note: Because this second phase of IFS therapy can release unpredictable pain, the healing steps are best learned in an official training.

Helping exiles is highly idiosyncratic and often surprising. In theory, this second phase of IFS therapy also takes place as a set of six steps that begin after re-establishing the trustworthy presence of Self: Witnessing, Do Over, Retrieval, Unburdening, Invitation, and Integration. These typically wrap up with an appreciation of all parts who participated. In practice, therapy often doesn't play out in a linear fashion. With a given client—and a given exile—some steps may not be needed and some may repeat, over and over. Because we follow the client's system in making decisions about how to proceed with healing, we may need to pay more or less attention to individual steps, depending on our own comfort levels and the client's needs. While it is important to help the exiles find relief, much of the work of IFS therapy is focused on helping the protectors be more trusting of the Self and its leadership within the system and, as a result, become less extreme in their protective behaviors—which, in turn, provides its own relief.

Re-establishing Trust

Just as the first stage of IFS therapy begins by helping protectors unblend, the second stage checks on and re-establishes a clear connection between Self and exiled parts. This involves checking for any Self-like protector parts that may have an agenda. Whenever it seems that protectors have come back in, we stop and acknowledge them with a gentle request that they step back so that Self can continue to lead.

By this point in the therapeutic process, we've already built a relationship of trust with our clients and our clients' protectors. Because exiles are particularly sensitive, we also check the level of trust between the Self and each exile by asking about preferences regarding proximity and contact. For a given exile, we might ask clients how close to/far from the part they are, and whether they may want to adjust the amount of separation. Can they get closer? Do they need more distance at first? We encourage the clients' Self to be in the lead, showing care, compassion, and openheartedness to the exile.

When protective parts are afraid that they'll experience the presence of the exiled part as overwhelming, we suggest that the client ask the exiled part in advance not to deluge the client with its complaints. When the request comes from the Self, and it is clear that it is intended to be helpful, exiles are often amenable to such an agreement. Because this step is an extremely important foundation for the rest of therapy, we want to take as long as necessary to build a caring relationship between Self and exiles.

If exiles are unresponsive or unwilling at first, we may need to negotiate with protectors and have a contract with them as we continue. For example, an exile carrying extreme anxiety may flood the system to such a degree that protectors and firefighters feel that they must jump in to restabilize it. Ideally, since we already know the protectors, we can ask them to step back enough for us to get to know the exile and its overwhelming anxiety, with the stated understanding that the protector will be there to witness the Self connecting to the exile. These delicate negotiations build trust in the Self for all the parts, no matter their roles in the system.

Step 1: Witnessing

Because exiled parts have been cut off, hidden, or pushed away, their primary need is to be seen, heard, felt, and understood—to no longer be alone. We help clients attune to their exiles, however they are expressing themselves by witnessing. Different parts may need different forms of expression to feel witnessed. Some exiled parts want to tell their stories, or share scenes from the past, in order to establish understanding. Other, seemingly "young," parts may not be verbally communicative, but may need to share the stuck feelings that they have endured alone by having the client feel and share their emotions and acknowledging their pain. Parts that have not been believed or have been denied usually need to use the body more to tell their story in order to feel fully understood. Witnessing needs to go at the pace of the exile, but as strong emotions are being expressed, if managers try to interfere, that's an indication that the process is going too fast and that you may need to cycle back to work with protectors.

Step 2: Do Over

Sometimes the process may go quickly; when there has been a great deal of trauma, it may take some time. In the witnessing step, we want to ask if "there's more" and have the client check to see if the part feels fully seen and understood. Sometimes the exile needs to reexperience the situation in the presence of Self offering the support that wasn't there in the past. IFS calls this a *do over*, an optional aspect of the healing steps sometimes framed as rescripting, that the therapist might offer during or after witnessing. When the client's Self is able to be fully present with the exiles' needs, exiles are no longer alone. When they are seen and heard by the compassionate Self, exiles become ready to shift. This step deepens and anchors the trust and internal attachment between the Self and the exile, so it's important that both the client and therapist have patience to stay with witnessing and do over until the exiled part feels satisfied.

Step 3: Retrieval

Exiled parts often feel stuck as if they are continuously, or repeatedly, reliving the experiences and feelings that caused their exile in the first place. That's why, when feelings are triggered in the present, they're experienced with such intensity: A minor current event may cause an outsized reaction because the exile is responding as if the event is occurring *in another time and place,* an ongoing world of painful memories, feelings, or possibilities in which the part has become stuck. Only after the client's Self has witnessed, experienced, and acknowledged the exile, frozen in time or place, can the Self bring the exile out of that painful experience and retrieve it from the immutable past.

Retrieval from the place or time where the part is stuck may emerge as a natural extension of witnessing, or it may need to wait until the part has released its burdens, which means that sometimes steps 3 and 4 may naturally exchange places. Following the client's lead, the IFS therapist asks the exile if it wants to be somewhere else, if it is ready to leave the bubble of the past or the stuck place and come into the present. If it does, Self can facilitate the return. Simply inviting an exile to come into current reality is often a powerful move in which the exile, in contact with Self, realizes that it is possible to leave the past behind. If the part is not ready or interested, we ask it what needs to happen first. It may be that protectors still have concerns, or perhaps the exile is connected to other parts that need attention first.

With the accompaniment and help of the Self, the client can update the part, orienting it to the mutable reality of the present. In this shift, Self in the current place and time becomes a secure connection to reality for the part that has continued to feel as if things endure as they used to be. While this re-established connection often happens happily and spontaneously, it's important to continue to check that Self-like protective parts are not being triggered and the client's Self is genuinely in the lead.

Step 4: Unburdening

When the time is right, usually after an exiled part has been fully witnessed and safely invited into the present, we ask the part what it's carrying that had caused the constriction and alienation. Encouraging the client to "just listen," we ask what messages, beliefs, and feelings the exile has taken on from circumstances, experiences, or messages. Often, we will hear about feelings of shame, of being bad, of being unlovable, or of being "too much" or "not enough." In what may seem like a leap of faith to the protective parts, we ask the exile what it would be like to let go of these beliefs, to let go of the intolerable feelings of fear, shame, or guilt. We guide the client's Self to ask the exiled part if it is ready to unload these burdens or release some of what it's been carrying.

There are many ways to support this process as it unfolds, but it's important for the therapist to trust the client's Self and to follow its lead. We may offer suggestions such as inviting the part to notice where the burden is felt in the body and allowing it to fall away, using the breath to let the burden go, or visualizing its departure. Often just the suggestion that it's possible to let go of a constricting belief is liberating, and much of the burden is released on the spot. Sometimes, however, the client's protectors and exiles have concerns about how to live or who to be without the burdens, so we hear those concerns and help the parts that are carrying them first.

The experience of unburdening can be quiet or quite emotional. It can occur as one big cathartic release or as a slow unfolding. As therapists, our role is to lend the confidence and compassion of our own Self to the process, to be present and support a sense of security in which we can hold open this space of possibility with the client. When the process seems complete for the moment, we check to see if the part has unloaded all the burdens or if there are more, and if so, what needs to happen next.

Step 5: Invitation

When an exile's constraining beliefs and feelings are gone, leaving an empty space that the burdens once filled, it's important to offer the possibility of inviting back the qualities and capacities that had been silenced and sidelined. Perhaps creativity was squashed by shame, for example; in that case, we might invite the qualities of play and curiosity back into the system and help the client reconnect with abandoned creative activities. Perhaps sociability was squashed by fear of the unknown; now we can invite the quality of confidence back into the system and help the client connect to a new community, class, or organization. Again, we do not make suggestions, but offer an invitation. We might ask, "What qualities were pushed out by the burden? What qualities would this part like to invite back in going forward?" Invoking a vision of a future that includes the positive qualities and capacities that have been constricted is important.

Step 6: Integration and Appreciation

Bringing the parts that have been exiled back into the system should be done mindfully and with care. The first step is to ask the unburdened part or parts what they would like to do now, where they would like to stay. We also ask the part what it would like from the client's Self going forward. Usually, it's advisable to encourage the client to check in with unburdened parts regularly for at least three weeks to anchor the change and the connection. After asking clients if they can make a realistic commitment to follow through with such check-ins, we support them in finding the best way to make this happen—to help them inhabit a balanced, Self-led system of parts, working together as a collaborative, balanced, and harmonious team.

The final part of this final step is to check back with the initial situation that activated the exile to see how the system has responded, updating the protectors as necessary so that they know what has happened. We invite them to recognize that Self has helped this exiled part unload its painful burdens, and to accept that this vulnerable part, along with its gifts, can now rejoin the Self and the whole system of parts in the present. We check in to acknowledge the protectors' reactions, thoughts, and concerns, if any, and to see what *they* would like to do now.

In wrapping up this work it's important to help clients consciously appreciate all of the parts that have relaxed, paused, or stepped aside to allow healing to happen. By recognizing their efforts, we are solidifying, for the client's whole system, the realization that healing was possible and that Self was always there to lead and offer a compassionate and confident presence throughout. We may suggest to clients that they circle back and notice any protective parts that had been skeptical or concerned, thanking them for their willingness to allow healing to happen. Such healing might not be what the protective parts expected; they may be surprised that an exiled part could be known and felt without overwhelming the whole. Appreciation rewards their trust, and the courage that it took for them to trust is acknowledged as well.

Methods Used in IFS Therapy

Many clients find themselves easily able to unblend from their parts once they realize that instead of *being* parts, they *have* parts. Because they now understand that they have access to more than one perspective internally, they can just ask a part to unblend. However, many others do not have that easy experience: Their protectors are so familiar and strong that they feel as if they are Self. In these cases, IFS therapists use additional techniques to help clients access some perspective.

Tracking and Mapping Protector Interactions and Relationships

Especially in complex cases, IFS therapists are interested in the multiple internal systems that make up a client's inner landscape; this includes the client's whole system, not just the problem parts called symptoms. As discussed in Chapter 1, our individual parts, like distinct family members, represent our many capacities and embody our personality traits. They also engage in alliances, and polarizations: dynamic relationships that grow and change and influence each another—including, for example, internal dyads that pair up, parts that are averse to one another, and parts that can become very cliquey and mean, causing others to live on the fringes or be exiled entirely. As previously mentioned, although it's natural that many, if not most, parts of a person are collaborative, working together to contribute their strengths toward valued activities and life goals, it's also natural for parts to disagree, have different perspectives, and sometimes work in opposite directions to counterbalance one another. Learning about the client's internal relationships is a useful way to get to know the client's inner landscape.

Externalizing Methods for Facilitating Unblending

Because IFS therapists are interested in a client's whole system, it can be challenging to keep track of a client's list of players. Externalizing parts is a great way to help clients both disidentify from their parts and relate to them differently. Therapists have always used various forms of externalizing methods: for example, drawing, playing with puppets, manipulating sand trays, and using chairs or other objects to represent parts. Externalizing is particularly useful for facilitating distance between two parts that may be polarized. For some clients, being able to visualize parts externally creates a huge shift that can be used to remind them to connect with their parts in-between sessions. Finding an object in the room to represent a part and having the client imagine the part in an empty chair are fairly standard methods of externalizing parts.

Mapping Parts

Especially in complex cases, IFS therapists create maps, both for ongoing tracking of the whole system and as an in-session method for helping clients unblend and access Self, especially when the client has a lot of parts showing up or is shifting from part to part. Mapping can involve any method we may use to represent parts and their relationships with one another. The simplest method is to name parts and put them on paper spatially, representing how close they are to one another and the nature of their relationship, that is, alliance or polarization. If there is another part that comes up with a feeling about the one on the page, we add that. Observing the parts on the page can have a palpable clarifying effect.

Conference Table and Variations

When many parts show up at one time, or when multiple parts have very different opinions, needs, or jobs, a useful technique for externalizing parts involves suggesting to clients that they slow down and imagine that various parts that are vying for attention are sitting around something like a conference table. (We adapt this method to the personal life experiences of individual clients by suggesting that, for example, they imagine their parts in a huddle with Self as a quarterback, on a stage with Self as the director, in a concert hall with Self as the conductor, etc. The idea is to help clients choose a relatable image so that they can begin to see their parts as members of a team and Self as the leader.) If they are visualizing themselves at the table as the one in charge, gently point out that this may be a *helper part*—a part with an agenda to improve the person in some way—that has shown up and suggest that the client ask it to move to the side so that Self can simply be present.

The conference table exercise can lead to better differentiation between Self and parts, as well as differentiation among parts so that each is able to see the intentions and concerns of the others under the guidance of the secure Self, who accepts them all and provides leadership that involves the whole system.

Insight and Direct Access

IFS therapy offers a variety of ways to connect with and communicate with parts depending on the client's ability to access Self. Two methods are *insight* and *direct access*. In the first method, the client's Self engages with the part. In the second method, the therapist's Self speaks to the part either implicitly or explicitly. These are essentially different avenues for exploring the 6 F's.

Insight

If clients are able to unblend and maintain a sense of differentiation from a given part, it is ideal to facilitate clients' own internal communication with their parts. Using the insight approach, the therapist guides or suggests that the Self-led client speak with the part. We might say something like, "Ask the angry part if it has a job, and—without thinking too much—just listen to what comes to mind." The goal is to help the client's Self become the guide and attachment figure for parts to learn to trust. The therapist guides, not directs, in order to support the conversation that the client's Self wants to have with protectors. The more internal trust the client develops in this way, the easier it becomes for the protective parts to relax and allow access to the exiled parts that need help.

Direct Access

When a part refuses to unblend, and the client's Self is not available to speak with the part, the therapist can still continue the conversation by addressing the part directly. Therapists use direct access—in either an implicit or explicit form—when clients are absorbed in the feelings of a part and overly identified with its perspective. In *implicit direct access*, therapists bring their own Self to the conversation with a client's part without calling attention to the fact. While most therapeutic modalities operate using this method to some extent, in my experience IFS brings more awareness to both sides of this communication process: reminding therapists to become aware of their own parts—so they can be more Self-led—as they help the client's parts make room for Self. In this way, we dramatically increase the impact of the therapy.

In *explicit direct access*, by contrast, therapists speak overtly to a part. We might say, "Can I speak to the part of you who calls you names?" Doing so brings an experience of the therapist's Self-energy to the part, modeling how the client's Self-energy could one day be used in a similar way to address an activated part. The reassurance, care, and trust the part may feel when being addressed directly by the therapist has the calming and soothing effect necessary to help the part trust more in Self-leadership; this trust can be transferred to the client's Self over time. Additionally, as clients witness such a conversation, they often gain perspective and can differentiate from the part to carry on the conversation from Self.

A Word on the Art of IFS Therapy

Although there is a fundamental process and flow to the IFS model, there is also an art to IFS. Rarely do things progress in a linear fashion, so our guiding principle as IFS therapists is to slow things down so that our clients can notice parts and differentiate from them. Whenever possible, we follow where the clients' systems need us to go, staying close to their experience. We trust that what our clients report in the present moment will guide us to where the focus needs to move in the next moment. Grounded in true curiosity, the IFS process enables all clients to engage in self-inquiry safely because it is not in the service of storytelling or other agendas.

IFS therapy trains therapists to notice their own parts, fostering a clear and strong presence that instills confidence in clients as they face their difficult feelings. When clients are unable to access Self, or are highly blended with parts, we substitute temporarily as the Self of their systems and use our experience to promote unblending and ensure the emotional and physical safety of the client as a first priority. If particularly challenging protective parts show up, we respond with confidence and help those parts trust that there is hope. By acknowledging all parts with compassion, we embody a courageous, welcoming stance that helps our clients find and access the tools they already have in order to create and secure lasting change.

Note

1 Sometimes clients are uncomfortable with "parts language," even outright rejecting it. While it can be productive to explicitly discuss IFS terminology with clients, it's primarily important to stay as close as possible to their own descriptions of their experience, letting their reports guide our discussions. If a client reacts negatively to the word "part," and not the underlying concept, there are many other ways to describe the experience. We can, for instance, refer to a part as "that state of mind" or the "voice that tells you …"

References

Schwartz, R. C., & Sweezy, M. (2020). *Internal family systems therapy* (2nd ed.). The Guilford Press.

Sweezy, M. (2023). *Internal family systems therapy for shame and guilt*. The Guilford Press.

Part II

What to Know about OCD

Chapter 3

An Overview of OCD

Although descriptions of people with obsessive-compulsive disorder (OCD) date back to the 14th century (Luibheid & Russell, 1982), we still do not entirely understand its causes or how best to conceptualize its phenomenology. Like other mental health syndromes, OCD is multifactorial. It is experienced psychologically, but various physiological components make it clear that OCD is rooted in the brain–body system. First, genetic research has demonstrated extremely high heritability: between 45% and 60% for child-onset OCD and between 30% and 40% for adult-onset OCD (Mahjani et al., 2021). A recent study identified a total of 25 credible causal genes (Strom et al., 2025). This genetic predisposition is cited as the reason that psychosocial triggers such as stress and trauma may lead to OCD in some people, but not in others. Second, research on Pediatric Acute-Onset Neuropsychiatric Syndrome and its subtype, Pediatric Autoimmune Neuropsychiatric Disorder Associated with Strep, has shown that OCD can also be triggered by infectious, environmental, and metabolic triggers (Swedo et al., 2015). In addition, a misdirected immune response that causes inflammation in the brain—a form of basal ganglia encephalitis—can lead to OCD symptoms. The fact that those symptoms respond to intravenous immunoglobulin, as well as to anti-inflammatory, steroid, and antibiotic treatments, sheds light on some of the challenges we face in understanding OCD. It is therefore essential not to diminish, underestimate, or misrepresent the brain–body nature of OCD in this discussion, even as we look at it from a new angle.

A Brief History of OCD

OCD is a neuropsychiatric disorder defined by the *DSM-5*—the American Psychiatric Association's *Diagnostic and Statistical Manual of Mental Disorders, Fifth Edition* (2022)—as the presence of obsessions and compulsions that are recurrent and unwanted, that interfere with daily functioning, and that are severe enough to require more than an hour a day to execute. It is a multigenic disorder tied to hyperactivation of the orbitofrontal cortex involving persistent thoughts about threat and harm, and it involves serotonergic, dopaminergic, and glutamatergic components (Pittenger et al., 2011).

Obsessions are intrusive and unwanted internal experiences (thoughts, feelings, sensations, urges, and/or images) that provoke anxiety and distress. *Compulsions* are internal or external behaviors (e.g., counting or handwashing) that people engage in to prevent or reduce anxiety and distress generated by an obsession. For our purposes, it's helpful to think of OCD as a collection of internal, recurring states of mind that are sparked by the intrusion of an obsession and that generate enough doubt, fear, and distress to lead to patterns of unwelcome behaviors that can be time-consuming, stressful, and counterproductive. These behaviors are highly idiosyncratic and fall into a variety of subtypes, making OCD complex and highly varied in its presentation.

OCD symptoms are exacerbated when the solutions people devise to relieve doubt and fear (i.e., compulsions) inadvertently create a cyclical process in which the temporary effectiveness of these neutralizing strategies reinforces the frequency and intensity of future obsessive intrusions. Once an *OCD cycle* begins, it escalates over time so that people's very efforts to protect themselves from obsessional anxiety and pain become the cause of even greater despair.

When left untreated or treated inappropriately, OCD tends to get worse, becomes increasingly entrenched, and can develop into a severe, chronic, and sometimes disabling disorder. It typically takes anywhere from 11 to 17 years for a person with OCD to be properly diagnosed and get access to effective care (Ziegler et al., 2021). Multiple studies have found that "as many as 40% of individuals qualifying for an OCD diagnosis have never received any treatment at all" (Szymanski, 2012). Due to this devastating state of affairs, symptoms for many people can be so severe that the World Health Organization has identified OCD to be the tenth leading cause of disability worldwide (Veale & Roberts, 2014).

Research has repeatedly found that the *mechanism* that drives OCD is neurologically mediated and best explained by brain research, whereas the *content* of OCD is psychologically and experientially derived (Radua & Mataix-Cols, 2009). Understanding this relationship provides clarity that facilitates both high-quality treatment and compassionate care for individuals with OCD as it provides the rationale for acknowledging both the disorder and the individual afflicted by it.

Data from brain-imaging studies suggests that each of the OC symptom dimensions is based on overlapping brain-based *alarm systems* that have the potential to become dysregulated due to genetic vulnerability, adverse environmental change during the course of development (maladaptive learning leading to brain changes), or brain injury. Viewed in this light, the simple existence of diverse mental states is not in itself pathological. They become pathological only due to the distress they cause, their persistence, and their tendency to occupy time to the exclusion of more normal activities (Leckman et al., 2005).

As a multifactorial disorder, the *content* of OCD's obsessions and compulsions is psychologically mediated through people's experiences, their background and family context, and their values, fears, and beliefs. The more a particular content area matters to a person, the more likely it is that OCD will make that content a focus of obsessions. Whereas intrusive thoughts are normal and experienced by roughly 90% of the population without distress (Shafran, 2006), people with OCD may appraise these thoughts differently (e.g., as dangerous), and then seek to eliminate or avoid them, inadvertently reinforcing their occurrence and the anxiety that accompanies them. Content is the most culturally variable aspect of OCD, as values and beliefs are highly contextual. Since OCD typically latches onto whatever a person values, it can develop around extremely idiosyncratic material or culturally reinforced themes such as religion and morality.

Because OCD is both a brain-based disorder and a pattern of learned behavior rooted in highly variable life experience, the content of a person's obsessions is specific to that person and rooted in fears rather than realities. To date, most research and empirically derived treatment approaches have been focused on the mechanics of OCD, which are presumed to be relatively consistent from person to person. However, because the themes of OCD are personal and idiosyncratic, truly effective treatment that goes beyond mere symptom reduction must take into account both biological *mechanisms* and psychological *content*, ensuring that treatment is tailored to each person's unique makeup and background. This makes the *experience-near* approach of Internal Family Systems (IFS)—one in which we listen closely to the experience of parts from their perspective—a valuable addition to traditional modalities of therapy for OCD.

Recent research on neuroplasticity offers many paths for reshuffling the neural connections in the brain. Functional magnetic resonance imaging studies of the impact of cognitive behavioral therapy on OCD show changes in glucose metabolism in significant regions of the brain, including decreased activity in previously overactive circuits and increased activity in regions associated with reappraisal and reductions in negative emotions (Saxena et al., 2009). Regardless of its etiology, clinical OCD is associated with hyperactivation of the frontal-striatal region of the brain (Leckman et al., 2010). This part of the brain has a low threshold for being triggered by possible danger. It doesn't take much to provoke doubt and obsessional fears, as well as the urge to perform compulsive rituals to reduce those fears. As we strive to improve treatment options, our goal is to intervene in the processes that drive compulsive behaviors at the expense of functional and valued activities.

Because 21–25% of the general population acknowledges having obsessions and compulsions (Fullana et al., 2009), yet clinical OCD is diagnosed in only 2–3% of the population worldwide (Rosenberg et al., 2005), it is therefore highly likely that therapists will encounter clients who report experiencing obsessions and compulsions of some sort, whether they have a psychiatric diagnosis or not. In some cases, clients will need a medication intervention, a treatment option that should always be considered when OCD is severe, but medication alone will not address patterns of learned behavior or provide clients with an opportunity to live a fuller life.

OCD Obsessions and Compulsions

A few decades ago, people defined obsessions and compulsions in terms of their *form*: Obsessions were viewed as *thoughts* (which happened internally) and compulsions were believed to be *actions* (behaviors that could be seen by others). For example, obsessive thoughts about harm would result in an action like *checking*—for instance, physically getting up and going back to a door numerous times to be sure it's locked. If no overt action occurred, it was believed that no compulsion existed. This led to the term "Pure O" or "purely obsessional" OCD.

Current conceptualizations of OCD have expanded and modified the scope of the definitions of obsessions and compulsions. Obsessions aren't limited to thoughts; they may also occur as feelings, sensations, images, or urges. Compulsions can involve both external and internal actions or behaviors. So, a thought that provokes anxiety is an obsession; a thought that responds to the obsession by reducing anxiety is a compulsion—for example, an individual who experiences an intrusive image of harm coming to a family member (obsession), and then compulsively engages in self-reassurance or a mental review of the precautions to take to keep family members safe (compulsion). Instead of identifying obsessions or compulsions by the form that they take, we now identify them according to their *function*.

Obsessions

Obsessions are intrusive, persistent, and repetitive thoughts, images, and urges. Experienced as unwanted, inappropriate, disturbing, and typically anxiety provoking, they are *ego-dystonic*: They feel like "not me." As our understanding of OCD evolves, conceptualizations can change. Whereas the predominant view is that obsessions are involuntary intrusions, they are also described as inferences of doubt (Aardema et al., 2005). Either way, there's a moment when an unbidden thought, image, or impression comes up, seemingly out of nowhere; it does so again and again, causing a great deal of distress. This is an obsession.

The content of obsessions can spring from a limitless array of concerns, but tends to fall into subtypes or themes in the following categories:

- contamination by physical content and/or emotional associations;
- fixation on responsibility for harm, bad luck, or other situations in which injury may occur;
- need for symmetry, order or a "just right" feeling;
- preoccupation with unacceptable or taboo thoughts, usually aggressive, sexual, or blasphemous in nature; and
- miscellaneous obsessions focused on uncertainty and discomfort and the need to know.

Details on each category follow in Chapter 4.

Individuals with OCD might become preoccupied by bodily sensations that they are convinced are proof of being dirty—even though they just washed their hands. They might repeatedly have the experience of disturbing images popping into their heads, or a fear that they may somehow lose control of themselves and do something they would regret. Functionally, obsessions stir up uncertainty, anxiety, and fear about potential catastrophic events, or feelings of disgust and other repellent feelings. Our minds' alarm systems are designed to get our attention when it is critical: It's their job to grab our attention and focus in on anxiety and discomfort as cues that we may be in danger. However, obsessions in OCD operate more like an overly sensitive car alarm that goes off with the slightest provocation.

Compulsions

Compulsions are repetitive behaviors, either mental or physical, that are intended to address the problem posed or created by the obsession. Their function is to eliminate, reduce, or control the unpleasant awareness, that is, to get the incessant sound of the alarm to stop. The compulsions that people develop to cope with their obsessions are as varied and personal as the obsessions themselves, and while the compulsive behaviors can be somewhat effective in the short term, they backfire in the long term. Individuals with OCD engage in compulsive behaviors meant to "fix" their obsessions. However, because they are treating a situation as dangerous ("I need to protect myself using these compulsive behaviors"), they are reinforcing their faulty alarm systems ("If you are trying to protect yourself, we really must have been at risk"). Because compulsive behaviors can reduce anxiety, but not fix the problem, they become self-perpetuating. The experience of some relief via the compulsive behavior is reinforcing and pulls individuals into cycles they can't break free from. Because the presence of these unintentionally reinforcing strategies is one of the key diagnostic features that differentiates OCD from other impulsive or addictive activities, recognizing them will be essential. There are four general types of compulsions.

Behavioral rituals, the most obvious of OCD compulsions, include a range of observable behaviors that can be elaborate or simple, practical or symbolic. These behaviors include but are not limited to checking, repeating or redoing, decontaminating, and ordering or arranging. Sometimes the discreet behavioral rituals are quite brief and may even be unrelated to the obsession, serving simply as a quick fix offering temporary relief from the obsession. Mini-rituals include actions such as wiping hands on pants to symbolize cleaning, squinting while looking at something to be sure that one is seeing it, and tapping or other tic-like behaviors.

Reassurance seeking is a type of compulsion that involves asking questions or making confessions or statements as a way of receiving reassurance and reducing anxiety. This reassurance is often sought from others, but self-reassurance can also be a quiet compulsion that, undetected, may undermine therapy. As opposed to questions or statements that genuinely seek information, the sole purpose of reassurance seeking is to reduce anxiety: "Tell me I'm not a horrible person." For instance, "It's not bad, right, that I hope my friend did bad on our science test?" a teen client might ask in a therapy session—or might just confess, "Today I was hoping my friend would fail our test." Whether questioning or confessing, the person wants to be reassured that it's OK to think such bad thoughts. While it's not helpful for the therapist to make a condemning response, neither is it helpful to refrain from condemning: both function as a reassurance. Sometimes, simply making a statement to see if the other person has a reaction provides enough relief. For instance, a teen client might say in a therapy session, "Today I was hoping my friend would do poorly on the science test." If we don't condemn such a thought, then the client feels relief about it and the compulsion is reinforced. This form of confessing provides implicit reassurance even if the person told says nothing. For this reason, reassurance seeking tends be the most pervasive undetected compulsion reinforcing OCD behind the scenes.

Mental rituals can go undetected for quite a while because they are not visible to others and are often misunderstood, and thus not reported, by the individual with OCD. They can be so brief as to be almost undetectable, such as a single word of self-reassurance or a mental "no" to negate an unacceptable thought. They may also be complex and cumbersome, for example a longer prayer or a review of an entire conversation. Repetitive mental processes designed to undo or neutralize a thought in an attempt to create the illusion of safety, or attempts to prove or figure something out (i.e., become more certain), are also considered mental compulsions.

Finally, *avoidance* perpetuates the OCD cycle by eliminating the experience of facing the sources of anxiety and discovering that it's manageable. Sometimes avoidance is a proactive behavior designed to prevent an OCD cycle; at other times, it's a response to dread that arises in anticipation of an event. Either way, avoidance perpetuates the OCD cycle by functioning as an anxiety-relieving behavior that interrupts a constructive response to an uncomfortable situation. For instance, some people with OCD avoid the anxiety of homework or hygiene-related tasks such as showering because they anticipate the ordeal of compulsions that will ensue. Other times the very thought of going somewhere evokes obsessive dread to the point that they avoid the outing altogether. The first response is an example of side-stepping anxiety with a pre-determined avoidance; the second is avoidance in reaction to obsessive fears.

The OCD Cycle

Obsessions and compulsions are the brain's attempt to protect a person from the experience of vulnerability to fear, doubt, disgust, guilt, shame, and/or uncertainty. The OCD cycle begins with a stimulus that triggers an obsession. Triggers can be *external*: people or places; things such as knives, bathrooms, and sweat; or the sight or sound of certain numbers and words. They can also arise *internally* as feelings, sensations, images, memories, or triggering thoughts. One particularly difficult thought occurs as a kind of self-fulfilling prophesy known as *thought–thought fusion*, in which the thought of possibly having an OCD thought becomes as triggering as having the thought itself. Triggers start the process, obsessions stir up anxiety, and compulsions provide short-term fixes. As the cycle repeats, these quick attempts to achieve peace become more and more extreme over time.

Paradoxically, by aiming to regain or ensure a *feeling* of calm or safety, obsessive doubt stirs up anxiety that prompts a compulsion to fix or neutralize the discomfort, thus momentarily achieving the goal—and it looks like the problem has been "fixed." However, when anxiety is responded to in this way, the person comes to believe that compulsions are the sole route to regain calm. Not only do compulsions confuse the individual about how to effectively solve the "problem," but they also function to exacerbate future obsessions and anxiety—trapping the person in a never-ending cycle.

Relying on compulsions interferes with the development of more functional capacities to self-regulate, tolerate anxiety, and cope with adversity, so a person with OCD becomes incrementally and increasingly intolerant of anxious feelings and reliant on compulsive behaviors, believing anxiety to be dangerous—and something to be eradicated, not faced.

In the OCD cycle, a trigger sparks an obsession which stirs up distress. When there is enough distress, a compulsion is performed that provides temporary relief. In the long run, the OCD cycle increases distress. Left untreated, OCD escalates over time to the point where the compulsions begin to cause more pain than they alleviate—and the solution becomes the problem.

The Role of Family Accommodation in Maintaining the Cycle

OCD is maintained by the reliance on compulsions to reduce anxiety and distress. Often, because the compulsions that people with OCD perform don't feel like *enough*, they will urge those around them to abide by the rules and regulations of their compulsions. They will say: "Wash after you go outside; change clothes after doing the laundry; don't come in my room; wait until I finish ritualizing." And often, caring family members and friends accommodate their requests. Ironically, these well-intentioned gestures of reassurance can inadvertently exacerbate the OCD cycle, a behavior called *family accommodation* (FA), the term for the behaviors of loved ones who serve the same purpose as compulsions, that is, helping the person avoid or reduce the negative states stirred up by obsessions (Pinto et al., 2013). When others perform those compulsions for the person with OCD, distress is temporarily alleviated but the agency of the Self is bypassed and the OCD cycle is reinforced. FA has been shown in many studies to be negatively correlated with treatment outcomes (Lebowitz et al., 2016). Consequently, including family members in OCD treatment is often essential when treating children who have OCD.

FA complicates OCD in two ways. First, when family members agree to live according to the rules of OCD, their attempts to be helpful reinforce the OCD by sending the message that the person with OCD is *right* that the uncomfortable feelings should be avoided or eliminated. In turn, they are now reinforcing the short-term relief that keeps the OCD cycle going. Second, FA helps individuals with OCD experience their symptoms as more manageable. The family is making the situation more tolerable, which often keeps a person from seeking help until the disorder becomes severe.

Differentiating What *Is* and What *Isn't* OCD

OCD obsessions are very different from ordinary preoccupations, worries, or rumination. People speak casually about being "obsessed" with something of interest—a new food, a musician, or their quest to buy a new car—things that they avidly devote time to investigating. But clinical OCD obsessions and compulsions are never pleasant, fun, or engaging. They are also distinct from worries about real-life issues such as getting to work on time or repairing the roof; these types of concerns prompt a person to do something functional, such as setting an alarm or calling a roofing company, actions that solve a real problem and lead to functional relief. Worries such as these may feel uncomfortable, but they are not experienced as intrusive or dangerous.

Obsessions in OCD are fear cues with the added qualities of being repetitive, unwanted, and often highly unreasonable. While neurotypical people might reluctantly appreciate their worries because they encourage accountability, people with OCD are not pleased with their obsessions because the obsessions come unbidden, strike out of the blue, make them very uncomfortable, and then lead to equally uncomfortable and dysfunctional compulsions.

One comparison that can be useful for understanding the experience of those with OCD is to contrast an intrusive, repetitive mental experience common to neurotypical people, such as having a song stuck in their heads, with the experience of someone with OCD. Although it can be annoying to anyone when a seemingly random song keeps playing over and over in their heads (especially if they don't *like* the song), eventually they know the song will fade away. Even if it's there off and on for days, they probably don't care enough to actively spend time trying to get rid of it. Nor do they spend time wondering what it might *mean* that it was *that* song instead of another song, or whether the lyrics have some secret message intended specifically for them. They don't have a physical "fight, flight, or freeze" reaction to it, becoming flooded with fear or anger about it. They don't despair that anything they happen to be doing when the song pops into their minds will become contaminated or ruined by it—a sort of "wet paint" phenomenon where the negative feeling spreads to anything it touches.

In contrast, when someone with OCD suffers intrusions that replay themselves like a stuck song, they have difficulty just letting them be there until they go away. Instead of eventually subsiding on its own, the intrusive thought, memory, or image becomes magnified in importance. As protective parts of the individual with OCD attempt to engage with this obsession, they develop exaggerated questions and narratives about what the intrusion means and how important it is. For example, a person with OCD may wonder: *Why is that song, and not some other song, in my head? I must have some twisted need to break up with my partner. But I don't really want to do that. But am I sure about that? How do I know? Is he the wrong guy for me? But that can't be what's going on because I really miss him when he's gone. I could ask him if I've been loving enough and if he feels close to me. Maybe that would resolve the issue. I'm not the kind of person who just gives up on relationships so why did that song get stuck in my head? Does it mean....*

This intense focus on the intrusion, and the distorted interpretations accompanying it, stir up anxiety and a perceived need to get rid of the anxiety—at which point a reactive part jumps in with a compulsive behavior that it feels *must* be done to eliminate or get rid of the disturbance.

In OCD, the relief of feeling *done with it* (whatever "it" is) remains elusive. When OCD obsessions occur, they have a nagging and consuming quality that gets in the way of people just walking away and forgetting that something felt dangerous until they adequately *prove* to themselves that it isn't. People with OCD feel that nothing else can happen, that there can be no relaxation—and certainly no happiness—until the obsession is addressed, which is why it feels so compelling to do something about it. The qualities of the obsessions are different than the regular intrusive thoughts had by everyone, and so is their quantity and persistence.

People with OCD have common cognitive biases that we will later address as the activities of obsessional parts:

- they have an inflated sense of their own responsibility;
- they over-value the importance of their thoughts;
- they are excessively concerned about controlling their thoughts;
- they have an overestimated sense of the threat involved in not controlling them;
- they are perfectionistic; and
- they are intolerant of uncertainty (Stewart & Hu, 2010)

These tendencies exist on a spectrum, and what differentiates people with OCD from others who have ruminative thoughts is the extreme and absolute, black-and-white nature of their obsessional thinking. Someone who does not have OCD might feel excessively responsible or tend toward perfectionism or alarmism, but these tendencies are not experienced as necessary for survival.

Likewise, many people engage in regular rituals, superstitious acts, or everyday compulsive behavior without having OCD. The key is the element of flexibility and knowing how much is enough. For instance, many parents set up a bedtime ritual for their babies and young children. This can be a healthy way to develop good sleep hygiene and promote consistency. Unlike the behaviors that characterize OCD, this ritual is a choice and can be skipped without undue amounts of stress and anxiety. Many people knock on wood or say "drive safely" when loved ones leave the house. The same element of choice is true here; if you don't have OCD, you might feel weird if you realize that you didn't knock on wood, but it won't overcome you with anxiety or make you run off the field in the middle of a soccer game to find a tree, for instance. The overwhelming sense of "I have to," "no matter what," or "just one more time" characterizes the experience of a person with OCD.

Other intractable repetitive behaviors, such as gambling, shopping, or food rituals, should also be differentiated from OCD as they are *addictive* in nature: They start with a pleasant behavior that receives reinforcement. There is never anything fun or pleasant about compulsions. They are always performed to get rid of a bad feeling, not to keep feeling good.

What Is OCD?

Because OCD can be organized around most any topic, it can be hard to distinguish it from depressive rumination or general anxiety. Typically, the difference is that the obsessions in OCD are experienced as intrusive and ego-dystonic rather than as actual worries, concerns, or desires. For instance, someone who is depressed may ruminate about suicide and be emotionally drawn to the idea, whereas someone with OCD would experience suicidal thoughts as alarming and horrifying. Someone with Generalized Anxiety Disorder may worry about real-life concerns that feel understandable, even if exaggerated, and they do not attempt to neutralize or eliminate the thoughts, whereas someone with OCD may find their own obsessions strange and incomprehensible (*What if I want to harm my child?* or *Will I become lazy if I sit next to this "underreaching" student?*) and perform rituals to neutralize them.

With OCD, a person will usually have multiple areas of concern, and so if a person is solely focused on a body part, health issues, or body image and food, then the issue may not be OCD. Finally, the content of OCD may seem bizarre and delusional, even to the person suffering from it; the vast majority of people with OCD do not literally believe that their fears are rational even when they feel very real.

From an IFS perspective, OCD involves (1) an internal or external trigger that gets the attention of parts, (2) proactive protective parts that manage the trigger, make interpretations, and tell stories that stir up often intolerable amounts of fear and uncertainty with the intention of preventing catastrophe, and (3) reactive protective parts that, believing they have the only solution, perform compulsions to attempt to neutralize the threat and calm the fear even though the person with OCD has no desire to take that action and usually realizes that it's unnecessary.

Case Examples

To illustrate the complexities of OCD and the strategies IFS offers to treat it, we will follow the treatment of three individuals through the rest of the book, fictional characters with symptoms common to people with OCD. These case studies are meant to illustrate, for those not familiar with OCD, the many ways OCD can show up. They are not meant to be exhaustive or to present actual case material. In the chapters to come, we will walk through traditional approaches in the assessment and treatment of these clients: What worked and where they hit roadblocks. We will then demonstrate how the IFS for OCD approach can be useful in the treatment of OCD.

Meet Justin

Justin, a cisgender, gay, married graphic designer in his mid-40s, came to therapy because his life was becoming increasingly limited by his hesitation to leave his house. A "germophobe" and "afraid of pretty much everything," he feared bathroom germs, getting sick, and passing on an illness to others. He also feared mold and other contaminants, including fumes from pollutants such as gasoline and pesticides. He reported that his extensive and ritualized handwashing took hours a day and left his arms and hands red, chapped, and bleeding. He limited his outside activity because of a refusal to use public bathrooms, but reported that he was also afraid of the second bathroom in his own house. His fear of germs affected other parts of his home life as well and necessitated ritualized steps when doing chores such as laundry, cooking, or taking out the trash. He also spent a great deal of time trying to decide which chore to do first, noting how the contamination from one item may have spread to the others without a shower in between. Doubt plagued his day, and he often stopped to review his steps to make sure he had done his washing and decontaminating rituals properly. Once done, his rituals allowed him a moment of relief, but soon he began to worry about what his hands had touched, or he started to feel intrusive sensations of tingling that he interpreted as proof of recontamination, and his anxiety rose until he repeated the washing rituals.

Meet Aracelli

Aracelli, a young stay-at-home mother of two, worried about harm coming to members of her family, primarily her husband and her children—an 8-year-old boy and 11-year-old girl. She had intrusive thoughts and images that were highly disturbing, which she attempted to fix by being excessively safety conscious and careful about household cleanliness, food preparation and potentially dangerous cleaning products as well as medications, laundry, and driving. Ironically, the avoidant and over-protective actions caused her and her family members a great deal of distress. Aracelli realized this and felt shame about it, yet also expressed an inability to stop. Her experience of what she called "abject terror" at the thought of allowing her children to buy school lunches, made them angry, and her husband left a good job so that he could help out more at home. Aracelli also struggled with immobilizing perfectionism when planning holidays or engaging in hobbies or projects, and engaged in extensive researching to be sure of anything that caused her doubt—from health symptoms to directions or the best birthday party theme.

Meet Scott

Scott, an 18-year-old, first-year college student, entered therapy because he was having trouble in school. Although he had managed to navigate high school with excellent grades, Scott was finding that in his new college environment (without his family to reassure and support him), stress and anxiety were taking over his life. When we first met, he appeared to be extremely efficient, self-aware, and earnest in his search for a solution. But quickly his desperation became clear as he haltingly described the agonizing event that finally convinced him that he needed help. During midterms, he had found himself repeating his schoolwork, which was not unusual for him. But one night, he submitted, unsubmitted, and then resubmitted an essay five times over the course of several hours. When he finally finished, after midnight, he found that he couldn't go to sleep until he checked one more time to make sure that he hadn't plagiarized something or failed to cite a source. And then he checked again. And again. Each time he got out of bed to check his work, he thought "one more time" would do it. Each time, soothed and relieved, he got back in bed but couldn't sleep. Thoughts would pop up asking: *Was that second point original, or did I paraphrase it without a citation? Is my reference list really complete?* With more questions, I learned that Scott followed a similar process when he posted on social media. He would doubt whether or not he'd actually taken the picture he posted, whether the words were his own, and whether the thought was original. Other areas of repetition and checking involved his passion for the environment and making sure his every action was sustainable and ethical for the planet.

References

Aardema, F., O'Connor, K. P., Emmelkamp, P. M. G., Marchand, A., & Todorov, C. (2005). Inferential confusion in obsessive–compulsive disorder: The inferential confusion questionnaire. *Behaviour Research and Therapy*, *43*(3), 293–308. https://doi.org/10.1016/j.brat.2004.02.003

American Psychiatric Association (Ed.). (2022). *Diagnostic and statistical manual of mental disorders* (5th ed., text rev.). https://doi.org/10.1176/appi.books.9780890425787

Fullana, M. A., Mataix-Cols, D., Caspi, A., Harrington, H., Grisham, J. R., Moffitt, T. E., & Poulton, R. (2009). Obsessions and compulsions in the community: Prevalence, interference, help-seeking, developmental stability, and co-occurring psychiatric conditions. *American Journal of Psychiatry*, 166(3), 329–336. https://doi.org/10.1176/appi.ajp.2008.08071006

Lebowitz, E. R., Panza, K. E., & Bloch, M. H. (2016). Family accommodation in obsessive-compulsive and anxiety disorders: A five-year update. *Expert Review of Neurotherapeutics*, 16(1), 45–53. https://doi.org/10.1586/14737175.2016.1126181

Leckman, J. F., Mataix-Cols, D., & do Rosario-Campos, M. C. (2005). Symptom dimensions in OCD: Developmental and evolutionary perspectives. In J. S. Abramowitz & A. C. Houts (Eds.), *Concepts and controversies in obsessive-compulsive disorder* (pp. 3–25). Springer.

Leckman, J. F., Denys, D., Simpson, H. B., Mataix-Cols, D., Hollander, E., Saxena, S., Miguel, E. C., Rauch, S. L., Goodman, W. K., Phillips, K. A., & Stein, D. J. (2010). Obsessive-compulsive disorder: A review of the diagnostic criteria and possible subtypes and dimensional specifiers for DSM-V. *Depression and Anxiety*, 27(6), 507–527. https://doi.org/10.1002/da.20669

Luibheid, C., & Russell, N. (1982). *The ladder of divine ascent* (J. Climacus, Trans., pp. 211–213). Paulist Press; original work composed in the 6th/7th century.

Mahjani, B., Bey, K., Boberg, J., & Burton, C. (2021). Genetics of obsessive-compulsive disorder. *Psychological Medicine*, 51(13), 2247–2259. https://doi.org/10.1017/S0033291721001744

Pinto, A., Van Noppen, B., & Calvocoressi, L. (2013). Development and preliminary psychometric evaluation of a self-rated version of the family accommodation scale for obsessive-compulsive disorder. *Journal of Obsessive-Compulsive and Related Disorders*, 2(4), 457–465. https://doi.org/10.1016/j.jocrd.2012.06.001

Pittenger, C., Bloch, M. H., & Williams, K. (2011). Glutamate abnormalities in obsessive compulsive disorder: Neurobiology, pathophysiology, and treatment. *Pharmacology & Therapeutics*, 132(3), 314–332. https://doi.org/10.1016/j.pharmthera.2011.09.006

Radua, J., & Mataix-Cols, D. (2009). Voxel-wise meta-analysis of grey matter changes in obsessive–compulsive disorder. *British Journal of Psychiatry*, 195(5), 393–402. https://doi.org/10.1192/bjp.bp.108.055046

Rosenberg, D. R., Russell, A., & Fougere, A. (2005). Neuropsychiatric models of OCD. In J. S. Abramowitz & A. C. Houts (Eds.), *Concepts and controversies in obsessive-compulsive disorder* (pp. 213-232). Springer.

Saxena, S., Gorbis, E., O'Neill, J., Baker, S., Mandelkern, M., Maidment, K., Chang, S., Salamon, N., Brody, A., Schwartz, J., & London, E. (2009). Rapid effects of brief intensive cognitive-behavioral therapy on brain glucose metabolism in obsessive-compulsive disorder. *Molecular Psychiatry*, 14(2), 197–205.

Shafran, R. (2006). Cognitive-behavioral models of OCD. In *Concepts and Controversies in Obsesssive Compulsive Disorder* (p. 456). Springer.

Stewart, E., & Hu, Y.-P. (2010). Faculty of 1000 evaluation for obsessive-compulsive disorder: A review of the diagnostic criteria and possible subtypes and dimensional specifiers for DSM-V. *F1000- Post-Publication Peer Review of the Biomedical Literature.* https://www.academia.edu/87367390/Faculty_of_1000_evaluation_for_Obsessive_compulsive_disorder_a_review_of_the_diagnostic_criteria_and_possible_subtypes_and_dimensional_specifiers_for_DSM_V

Strom, N. I., Gerring, Z. F., Galimberti, M., Yu, D., Halvorsen, M. W., Abdellaoui, A., Rodriguez-Fontenla, C., Sealock, J. M., Bigdeli, T., Coleman, J. R., Mahjani, B., Thorp, J. G., Bey, K., Burton, C. L., Luykx, J. J., Zai, G., Alemany, S., Andre, C., Askland, K. D., ... Mattheisen, M. (2025). Genome-wide analyses identify 30 loci associated with obsessive–compulsive disorder. *Nature Genetics.* https://doi.org/10.1038/s41588-025-02189-z

Swedo, S. E., Seidlitz, J., Kovacevic, M., Latimer, M. E., Hommer, R., Lougee, L., & Grant, P. (2015). Clinical presentation of pediatric autoimmune neuropsychiatric disorders associated with streptococcal infections in research and community settings. *Journal of Child and Adolescent Psychopharmacology, 25*(1), 26–30. https://doi.org/10.1089/cap.2014.0073

Szymanski, J. (2012). Using direct-consumer marketing strategies with obsessive-compulsive disorder in the nonprofit sector. *Behavior Therapy, 43,* 251–256.

Veale, D., & Roberts, A. (2014). Obsessive-compulsive disorder. *BMJ, 348,* g2183. https://doi.org/10.1136/bmj.g2183

Ziegler, S., Bednasch, K., Baldofski, S., & Rummel-Kluge, C. (2021). Long durations from symptom onset to diagnosis and from diagnosis to treatment in obsessive-compulsive disorder: A retrospective self-report study. *PLoS One, 16*(12), e0261169. https://doi.org/10.1371/journal.pone.0261169

Chapter 4

Assessment and Diagnosis of OCD

Accurate assessment and diagnosis are key to the treatment of obsessive-compulsive disorder (OCD). There is collective trauma in the OCD community around the experiences of those who were not able to find help because of misdiagnosis and/or spent years in ineffective therapy. Obsessions are internal experiences that are sometimes subtle and often embarrassing; they may not be reported to therapists or recognized by them because the content areas of obsessional concerns, while infinitely wide ranging, are commonly reduced to the standard domains of contamination and symmetry. Mental compulsions are easy to miss or to label as distraction if you are not trained to recognize them, so children with OCD are commonly diagnosed with attention-deficit/hyperactivity disorder (ADHD). Conversely, it's also possible to improperly diagnose OCD where it *doesn't* exist. Some repetitive behaviors seen in addiction, impulsivity, or autism, for instance, may look similar to OCD, but they don't have the same neurological features and negative reinforcement cycles that cause OCD symptoms to become worse over time.

This chapter summarizes the relevant aspects of typical OCD assessment and the tools for proper diagnosis. It is intended to give clinicians who don't specialize in treating OCD enough information to screen for it and make appropriate clinical decisions. This chapter begins with a discussion of the need for accurate assessment and then presents some of the more common foundational assessment procedures. It continues with a discussion of OCD subtypes and concludes with initial assessments of the clients in our three case studies, demonstrating a basic application of these assessment procedures—and serving as a precursor to the introduction of Internal Family Systems (IFS) therapy for OCD in their cases, presented in Parts III and IV of the book.

Increasing Awareness about OCD

Although media coverage of OCD has increased, a lack of sound education about the disorder leaves many who experience it without the knowledge needed to understand their experiences and also leaves many therapists

DOI: 10.4324/9781003449812-7

without the tools to assess and diagnose it. Far too many individuals are newly diagnosed late in life adding grief and anger about lost decades to their list of issues to deal with in therapy.

Because OCD can get progressively worse if untreated or mistreated, learning to recognize it is important even if OCD is not your clinical specialty. When clients present with OCD, therapists should start by determining its range and its severity to decide whether they have the necessary expertise to treat it, and, if so, to what extent and in what ways they will do it. We may determine that IFS is a valuable initial approach to foster willingness and readiness for first-line exposure and response prevention treatment because IFS allows us to work with the parts of a client who are hesitant about or shutting down treatment and need help first. With skill, IFS may be used throughout treatment to work directly with the parts involved in the OCD cycle. Whether or not we ultimately use IFS with our clients who may have OCD, starting with a good assessment is critical.

Assessment of OCD

Accurate assessment allows us to meet clients where they are so that they can feel understood and that their parts are acknowledged. OCD can be difficult to assess informally because its manifestations are highly variable and shape shifting, and the specifics of its obsessions and compulsions are often so disturbing that clients may feel disinclined to share them. Many individuals may not recognize that their horrifying, intrusive thoughts are caused by a disorder, not a personal failing. As a result, they may be experiencing layers of shame leading to a tendency to hide. The therapist's ability to demonstrate familiarity with the nature of these disturbing obsessions can go a long way toward putting clients at ease.

That's why following a thorough OCD assessment process is valuable: It can result in a clear, evidence-based diagnosis that's communicable to clients. Often, receiving that diagnosis provides clients with an initial wave of relief because it offers them a destigmatizing explanation for symptoms, replacing the blame and shame they have experienced with a sense of validation ("This doesn't define me!") and normalization ("Other people are experiencing the same thing I am. I'm not alone.").

In addition to the symptomatic features of OCD, the many factors that contribute to the complexity of the disorder make it crucial to gather information about all aspects of a client's clinical picture. Although we may return to assessment time and again during therapy, the initial structured assessment of factors that affect clinical decisions about course of treatment with OCD proceeds in a roughly linear order. We begin by asking questions about the client's background and relevant family and medical history. Following *The Diagnostic and Statistical Manual of Mental*

Disorders, Fifth Edition (*DSM-5*) guidelines, we have the option of using one or more standard inventories to assess the client's kind and severity of OCD symptoms. We conclude this initial work by assessing the client's safety-seeking behaviors, prompts, and triggers, and the client's level of insight (Rapp et al., 2016, p. 21). Outside of the structured assessment, we may need to gather more detailed information about what drives and maintains the client's OCD. Triggers for OCD may evolve and the originally presented triggers may not be complete so more information should be collected and noted on an ongoing basis. The same is true of safety behaviors and avoidances that may become clearer as the therapy progresses.

Background and Relevant History

We gather family and medical history to understand the client's experience, including previous therapy attempts, medical issues, and psychiatric evaluations. OCD's high heritability (Van Grootheest et al., 2005) makes family history valuable for assessment. Key information includes onset age, duration without treatment, and previous interventions. Risk assessment covers not only self-harm and violence (typically low), but also physical harm from OCD behaviors (potentially high), such as restricted fluid/food intake or skin damage from excessive washing. These issues should be directly addressed as clients may not initially report them (Pampaloni et al., 2022).

Symptoms of OCD

Careful assessment of OCD balances the importance of an accurate diagnosis with the clinical needs of the partnership between therapist and client. Because OCD appears in many different forms and expressions, assessment appropriate to different individuals calls for different methods, some of which integrate with IFS better than others. From an IFS perspective, information from these assessments can be useful as an indicator of the extent to which the behavior of a protective part is causing problems.

The American Psychiatric Association's *DSM-5 TR* (2022) offers valuable guidelines for identifying OCD:

- Recurrent, unwanted, and intrusive thoughts (i.e., obsessions), and/or
- Repetitive behaviors or rituals (i.e., compulsions) that are intended to relieve the fear, anxiety, and/or distress associated with obsessions, and that are severe enough to require more than an hour per day to execute
- Obsessions and/or compulsions that cause significant distress and impairment in social, academic, and/or family functioning
- Symptoms that are not due to another disorder.

Structured assessment by means of standard OCD inventories can be completed at the beginning of therapy and then quickly and easily retaken at a later date to demonstrate to other parts that Self has become more present. They are important with OCD as a guide for therapy because hidden symptoms of OCD can sabotage progress.

An important category of symptoms often missed by common OCD inventories is safety-seeking behaviors, which include all actions, activities, and experiences, both mental and physical, that a person may avoid in the service of not triggering OCD. Clients often engage in safety-seeking behaviors in order to prevent or relieve strong feelings and may have come to accept the behaviors as normal adjustments to their lives, so it may not be until discussing the motivation for treatment or values that clients report on parts of their lives that are missing. A thorough assessment should therefore include questions that address whether or not clients are avoiding certain situations, people, hobbies they used to enjoy, friendships, etc. They may have not applied for certain jobs or school because of anticipated challenges and there may be life goals that are not even considered.

Severity of Symptoms

Assessing the client's functional impairment across social competence, adaptability, occupation, impulse control, emotional regulation, and decision-making is crucial. Standardized measures like the Yale-Brown Obsessive-Compulsive Scale (Goodman, et al., 1989) help quantify severity and inform treatment focus. The needs and deficits determined by means of this information will guide our decisions about referrals, the focus of the work, and the treatment approach we decide to employ.

Prompts and Triggers

Starting with the beginning of the assessment process, we take note of the items, thoughts, or situations that may spark the OCD cycle so we can help protective parts trust that we understand what drives them. These triggers include both external situations and stimuli that stir up protectors as well as internal events—such as bodily sensations or intrusive memories or images—that spur protectors into action. People with OCD tend to be highly attuned to minute, internal signals of danger such as changes in heart rate or tingling sensations or tightness in the chest or stomach—which may not even rise to the level of awareness and still spark obsessions.

Level of Insight

Studies demonstrate that patients with OCD who have poor insight show significantly worse treatment outcomes in a three-year prospective follow-up compared to those with good insight. Researchers have found that poor insight was associated with greater symptom severity, poorer response to both pharmacological and psychological treatments, and higher rates of relapse (Catapano et al., 2010; Jacob et al., 2014). This is an area in which IFS can have a beneficial impact on sufferers. When the obsessive-compulsive cycle becomes severe, a person may have very little ability for perspective taking and limited access to Self. In these cases, we can lean on the assessment tools offered by IFS (discussed in Chapter 9) noting the client's ability to develop Self-to-part relationships.

Clinical Applications

Choosing and administering the proper assessment strategy is an important part of the work with someone who may have OCD. Often it's the first time that individuals experience the destigmatizing impact of feeling understood and are able to gain access to self-compassion amid the hope that relief is on the way. During the assessment process, specific themes that are the focus of the client's OCD will usually come to light. These themes designate a subtype of OCD. Helping clients identify their subtypes as part of the early psychoeducation that naturally occurs in the assessment phase can increase their confidence in, and hope for, the therapeutic process.

Subtypes of OCD

OCD is known by clinicians and researchers to be a heterogenous syndrome, meaning that it has distinct, recognizable, and sometimes overlapping symptom dimensions and subtypes or themes. Although obsessions and compulsions are common to all types of OCD, their expression is highly individual and represents the many ways that a person's values and life experiences shape the disorder into a complex, highly refined, and effective form of torture. People with OCD can experience the obsessions and compulsions of more than one subtype, and their subtype(s) may change over time. In fact, no one universally agreed-upon set of subtypes exists; they are defined differently depending on whether their characteristics are discussed in a research, clinical, or general context.

For the purposes of this book, I categorize subtypes of OCD into five groups identified by their obsessional content and based roughly on the symptom checklists found in OCD inventories and other literature (Abramowitz & Jacoby, 2016): (1) contamination; (2) responsibility for harm; (3) symmetry, order, and "just right" obsessions; (4) unacceptable, intrusive thoughts, usually violent or sexual; and (5) a broad category of uncertainty-focused obsessions or "need to know" obsessions. A myriad of other clinical systems use more experience-near approaches to naming subtypes, identifying them by the obsessive theme, for example, Relationship OCD, Existential OCD, Pedophilia OCD, etc. I will use a combined approach that both captures the relatable naming of subtypes and maintains the integrity of thematic research.

It is notable that the subtypes of obsessions and the categories of compulsions (behavioral rituals, reassurance seeking, mental rituals, and avoidance) do not line up on a one-to-one basis. Compulsions may appear in any form and are always directly related to the obsessive content, although it may not be obvious to the observer how they are connected. Typically, contamination obsessions are paired with washing and checking compulsions, but they may also be soothed by reassurance or a magical tapping ritual, for example. Obsessions about responsibility for harm are most typically met by reassurance seeking and checking compulsions, but sometimes people may wash their hands to "clean" or "clear" the thoughts. Symmetry concerns are usually fixed by repeated ordering and counting, and taboo thoughts are most often eliminated by mental compulsions and reassurance seeking, but any effective ritual or safety behavior could be used. For that reason, we do not attempt to force obsessions and compulsions into combined subtypes, but allow the naturally mixing and matching with obsessional content as the overarching theme.

Contamination-Focused Obsessions

Contamination is the most well-known of the OCD subtypes, but it is not well understood. Contamination fear has two core dimensions, namely harm and disgust (Melli et al., 2015), and these are distinct from what is called emotional contamination. Some people with physical contamination OCD are worried that dirt, germs, viruses, chemicals, and other substances will make them sick or will lead to them being responsible for making others sick. Other people with physical contamination OCD feel that things are "dirty" or "contaminated" with something that evokes disgust. The triggers can include germs, bodily waste, hospitals and doctors, people and animals, or contaminated or expired food, toxins, and other environmental contaminants. They might also fear ingesting dangerous items such as broken glass, poisonous plants, medication, or things that are gross, including bodily fluids, sticky or greasy substances, and smears. It can be helpful to differentiate between things that are actually dirty, and things that *feel* dirty or are contaminated. Clarifying the language can help with both assessment and treatment interventions.

Another type, very common but less well known, is called emotional contamination. People experiencing emotional contamination are negatively affected by contact with an idea, a concept or by association with something they deem undesirable or unsavory. Clients may fear that contact with a person, place, object, or thought will contaminate them in a way that feels dangerous and highly threatening. Contact can include seeing a text from the "contaminated" person, hearing a voice, or seeing a sign with a word that is "unclean" or even simply knowing that a person has been in the house and may have sat in a chair. This possibility of contact stirs up fear that these associations will spread and alter one's personality or essence.

Harm-Focused Obsessions

Harm-focused obsessions center around feelings of responsibility and the need to protect oneself from feelings of guilt, shame, or the sense of being at fault or to blame for some perceived negative action. These obsessions focus on the desire to remove all doubt about whether something could have been the individual's fault. This need can range from mild to severe, and when guilt becomes present, the issue of retribution and punishment is not far behind. Responsibility for harm is an overarching category that can include many content areas; some overlap with the contamination and taboo subtypes. A common thread is fear of accidentally being at fault or failing to take necessary action to prevent bad things from happening to oneself or others. Another fear that often arises is that of having a harmful identity, of *being* someone who has these thoughts and might want to do these things—even though that sounds horrifying to the person. Sometimes there's an accompanying fear that thinking something is as bad as doing it, or that thinking it may cause an unconscious and uncontrollable urge to act that way. There is also a fear of losing control and engaging in harmful acts.

One very painful theme common in the category of Harm OCD is pedophilia-themed obsessions. Here the focus of the fear is on thoughts of acting in a sexual manner toward children and of having a harmful identity, of being someone who would even think about such a thing, which leads people to avoid anything that may trigger the thoughts. Reassurance-seeking compulsions (including self-reassurance) are common, as are self-punishing thoughts and behaviors such as looking up information to discriminate between oneself and those who are pedophiles.

Perinatal OCD is another common topic in Harm OCD, including fears that are focused on one's own child or children. Intrusive thoughts can be so disturbing that people may avoid holding their own infants. Compulsions frequently include checking and mental reviewing to be sure not to be neglectful or careless in any way.

Sometimes harm obsessions are of a smaller but more constant nature. They include daily worries about making mistakes, being responsible for inconveniencing others, hurting their feelings, or inadvertently insulting them. Manifestations here may include mental compulsions, such as repeatedly reviewing conversations to be sure nothing offensive was said.

Rightness, Symmetry, and Order-Focused Obsessions

These obsessions can seem very different from the usual thoughts because they are often described more as feelings or urges. The compulsions are designed to get rid of discomfort and protect from feeling wrong, off, or imperfect. This grouping of obsessions is often called "just right" OCD. Some people experience discomfort or agitation when objects are not lined up correctly, are asymmetrical, or are not in a perfect pattern. For instance, if an object is touched with the right hand, it must also be touched with the left. This type of obsession may also include completeness: If a project is started, it must be finished in the same session. People may also experience obsessions about perfectionism in maladaptive ways. They repeatedly wonder if others have understood them perfectly, want to know everything about a certain topic, or keep their home in perfect order.

"Just right" obsessions are often persistent sensations and feelings that something is off in any area of life. People experiencing a need for things to be "just right" think that if they can't achieve the right feeling, something bad will happen, or anxiety about something bad happening won't go away. "Just right" obsessions differ from perfectionism in that the end result—it feels right—might vary from time to time within the same ritual.

Unacceptable or Taboo Thoughts–Focused Obsessions

This category focuses on content deemed abhorrent by the person experiencing it. It involves shame and fear about possibly having qualities or even simply having thoughts that are offensive to one's own values.

Religious scrupulosity is the specific term used to describe the type of OCD in which people suffer from a fear of offending their religious figures (such as God). Moral scrupulosity describes extreme concerns about behaving in any, even the slightest, way that doesn't align with one's own morals or values. Both types of scrupulosity include preoccupation with, and excessive irrational fear of, having blasphemous or unethical thoughts and being caught and punished. People experiencing scrupulosity fear violating rules or norms, failing to be completely honest, or having the best possible intentions.

Some people have disturbing intrusive thoughts of an aggressive or sexual nature. They may be preoccupied with an excessive irrational fear of losing control and acting on an unwanted impulse to harm themselves or others or fear images in which they see violent content. People experiencing sexual obsessions have intrusive, unwanted, or disturbing thoughts about wanting to engage in, or losing control and engaging in, sexual behaviors, acts, and impulses that are undesirable or outside of their own ideas about the realm of acceptability.

It's important to note from an assessment perspective that what differentiates individuals with the OCD subtypes of Harm and Unacceptable Thoughts from those who may be having violent or self-harm ideation is that people with OCD are appalled by their own thoughts. The obsessions do not represent any real desire, but instead cause disgust, shame, and fear.

Need to Know – Focused or Intolerance of Uncertainty–Focused Obsessions

Needing to know for certain about any topic or question for which there are no concrete answers is a variety of OCD organized around eliminating all uncertainty. This type of OCD has many varieties; it can include fears focused on an individual's sexual orientation or gender identity that are not consistent with a person's actual sense of who they are, worry about having a severe physical or mental illness, and concerns about memory, mental faculties, or the passage of time. Here the discomfort is focused on the vague notion of "knowing for sure." These subtypes include obsessions where the central concern is protecting oneself from feelings of doubt and uncertainty, or from being unsure about any among a wide range of concerns.

Relationship OCD involves extreme and unwarranted uncertainty about various aspects of one's relationships, usually but not always romantic, which can include doubts such as whether one's partner is "the one" or if the love felt for that partner or child is "pure" or "right." It can also focus on aspects or qualities of the partner or the partner's past relationships or features of their appearance.

Existential OCD involves a vague sense of uncertainty about the meaning of life and one's purpose, doubts about one's reality, and, for example, whether or not we are, or exist within, a simulation. These obsessions can be highly disturbing and lead to primarily mental compulsions, including rationalizing, hypothesizing, and mental checking.

Hyperawareness OCD, sometimes called Somatic OCD when focused on the body, involves the fear that one will never stop noticing an aspect of oneself, such as a bodily sensation, position, or feeling. It can also include a state of mind or abstract personality features. Much of the focus with these obsessions is on whether or not the obsession will ever subside, which is why it is included in the uncertainty category.

Finally, magical obsessions include a focus on the possibility of something bad happening, having bad luck, or that encountering unlucky numbers, colors, words, or symbols, or having a bad thought, can cause the bad thing to happen. Compulsions involve behaviors such as knocking on wood or tapping or chanting mantras. Repetitive rituals may be performed to magically prevent bad things from happening and clean, clear, or reset a situation or a feeling.

Initial Assessments

Recognizing possible OCD is the first step toward helping clients release the grip that these obsessive and compulsive protectors can have on their lives. The earlier this diagnosis is made, the easier the release can be.

Justin's Initial Assessment

In our assessment, we learned that Justin struggled with bodily waste, and, by extension, laundry, garbage bins, germs from other people and their cars, doctors' offices, and all public places. Bathrooms were particularly challenging, even his own: He worried that an article of his clothing might touch something contaminated in his bathroom, that he might spread that contamination when he sat on or touched things in the house or public areas, and that the contamination would spread unknowingly to someone else. In order to minimize that possibility, he took his clothes off before using the bathroom. Because he avoided all public bathrooms, he therefore would not attend events that were likely to last all day.

Because of these factors, we can hypothesize that Justin suffered primarily from Contamination-focused OCD.

Aracelli's Initial Assessment

Aracelli had obsessions about harm coming to her husband, her children, or her pets. These included several content areas such as food preparation and child proofing. She worried, "If they choke on something they ate or get hurt at a friend's house it'll be my fault." These thoughts were often accompanied by intrusive images of a choking incident or, at other times, vivid imagery of her children lying dead in their beds. The images induced increasing anxiety, fear, and dread until Aracelli performed sufficient checking or mental review: for example, checking the blender to make sure the blade had not come off in the smoothie she made for them or making sure the lunch she prepared was safe. She would also get up in the middle of the night to make sure her children were still alive. She also avoided driving far from home and eliminated glassware and potentially toxic cleaning products from the house. Aracelli also had fears about losing things, leaving doors unlocked, and keeping cleaning products locked up. Another obsession involved a perfectionistic fear of hurting or disappointing them in other ways. She engaged in ritualized efforts to find them the ideal gifts or plan the perfect birthday party for instance.

Because of these factors, we can hypothesize that Aracelli suffers primarily from harm-focused OCD with some features of perfectionism.

Scott's Initial Assessment

Scott's obsessions with being a good person extended beyond his concerns about breaking rules. He was obsessed with citing other people's work when writing, failing to act in accordance with his values about environmental concerns, and treating others, particularly women, with respect. He doubted his own good intentions if he spent time with people who didn't share these values, and considered distancing himself from people he saw drinking from plastic water bottles. His food intake was severely limited by ethical concerns, choosing to eat only organic, locally sourced, and eco-friendly vegan food. When those options were unavailable, he was wracked with guilt, unless he opted not to eat at all. Scott's obsessive doubt about whether or not he was being the best possible person manifested as a cruel voice in his head taunting him with thoughts like *What kind of person wouldn't just check? It's the least you can do!* Other compulsions included keeping his distance from women while walking to class and avoiding eye contact with them for fear of making them feel uncomfortable.

Because of these factors, we can hypothesize that Scott suffers from unacceptable thoughts – focused OCD, primarily moral scrupulosity.

Next Steps

Most IFS clinicians don't specialize in treating OCD, but that doesn't mean we can't learn to recognize its symptoms or make good decisions about how best to help. Even if the ultimate decision is to refer out, the first step is understanding that OCD is far more than the stereotypical washing and checking presented in mainstream media; it's a multifaceted and dynamic constellation of symptoms that includes both distress-inducing obsessions and compulsive relief-seeking thoughts and actions. Once we determine that our clients are in the grips of OCD, we can utilize the principles of the powerful and effective, evidence-based treatment methods for OCD within the compassionate and experiential paradigm of IFS to facilitate healing and stop the cycle.

References

Abramowitz, J. S., & Jacoby, R. J. (2016). *Obsessive-compulsive and related disorders: A guide for clinicians*. Oxford University Press.

American Psychiatric Association (Ed.). (2022). *Diagnostic and statistical manual of mental disorders: DSM-5-TR* (5th ed., text revision). American Psychiatric Association Publishing.

Catapano, F., Perris, F., Fabrazzo, M., Cioffi, V., Giacco, D., De Santis, V., & Maj, M. (2010). Obsessive-compulsive disorder with poor insight: A three-year prospective study. *Progress in Neuro-Psychopharmacology and Biological Psychiatry, 34*(2), 323–330.

Goodman, W. K., Price, L. H., Rasmussen, S. A., Mazure, C, Fleischmann, R. L., Hill, C. L., Heninger, G. R., Charney, D. S. (1989). The Yale-Brown Obsessive Compulsive Scale: I. Development, use, and reliability. *Archives of General Psychiatry, 46*(11):1006–1011. https://doi.org/10.1001/archpsyc.1989.01810110048007

Jacob, M. L., Larson, M. J., & Storch, E. A. (2014). Insight in adults with obsessive-compulsive disorder. *Comprehensive Psychiatry, 55*(4), 896–903.

Melli, G., Chiorri, C., Carraresi, C., Stopani, E., & Bulli, F. (2015). The two dimensions of contamination fear in obsessive-compulsive disorder: Harm avoidance and disgust avoidance. *Journal of Obsessive-Compulsive and Related Disorders, 6*, 124–131. https://doi.org/10.1016/j.jocrd.2015.07.001

Pampaloni, I., Marriott, S., Pessina, E., Fisher, C., Govender, A., Mohamed, H., Chandler, A., Tyagi, H., Morris, L., & Pallanti, S. (2022). The global assessment of OCD. *Comprehensive Psychiatry, 118*, 152342. https://doi.org/10.1016/j.comppsych.2022.152342

Rapp, A. M., Bergman, R. L., Piacentini, J., & Mcguire, J. F. (2016). Evidence-based assessment of obsessive–compulsive disorder. *Journal of Central Nervous System Disease, 8*, JCNSD.S38359. https://doi.org/10.4137/JCNSD.S38359

Van Grootheest, D. S., Cath, D. C., Beekman, A. T., & Boomsma, D. I. (2005). Twin studies on obsessive–compulsive disorder: A review. *Twin Research and Human Genetics, 8*(5), 450–458. https://doi.org/10.1375/twin.8.5.450

Chapter 5
Evidence-Based Treatment Options for OCD

In 1966, the first successful treatment for obsessive-compulsive disorder (OCD) was documented when psychologist Victor Meyer introduced a behavioral technique that he called exposure and response prevention (ERP) therapy, which he conducted with two individuals who experienced relief (Foa et al., 2012; Meyer, 1966). Starting with manageable situations, Meyer had his patients confront anxiety-producing situations without ritualizing and instructed them to stay with the anxiety until it naturally dissipated. The innovative aspect of his technique was combining exposure with actively preventing the compulsive response; previous treatments had tried exposure alone or other approaches but hadn't systematically prevented the rituals.

Prior to Meyer's discovery, recovery from OCD was considered impossible: Therapeutic interventions including psychodynamic psychotherapy, operant-conditioning procedures, and a wide variety of medications had all been unsuccessful. Now we know that a significant number of people (60–80%) who complete ERP therapy experience a substantial reduction in symptoms and are able to maintain those gains over time (Abramowitz, 1998; Foa et al., 2012; McKay et al., 2015). Given the dramatic turnaround in prognosis for people with OCD since the discovery of exposure therapy, it's important for anyone treating clients with the disorder to be familiar with the underpinnings of ERP, so that we can understand and effectively incorporate its beneficial principles into our therapeutic practice.

Still, while ERP is highly effective in treating many individuals with OCD, it also has limitations. Some individuals, for one reason or another, do not respond to ERP and need something more. My goal is to highlight the similarities between ERP and Internal Family Systems (IFS) and unite their strengths to develop a complementary model. Using IFS in the treatment of OCD, with a method I call Self-led ERP, may provide options for clients who haven't benefited fully from traditional ERP alone.

As discussed in Chapter 3, OCD has multiple, interconnected bases in biology, neuroanatomy, learning, and experience. When we understand

DOI: 10.4324/9781003449812-8

that OCD occurs at the intersection of brain and behavior, it becomes clear why the "talk therapies" of the early 20th century failed: They often served only to reinforce the mentally compulsive aspects of OCD without accessing the mechanisms needed for real transformation. Behavioral approaches, medication intervention, and the combination of the two have made a significant impact, improving many lives.

This chapter reviews the empirical foundations of exposure-based treatments as a foundation for readers who are new to treating OCD and to set up our discussion in Chapter 8 of how IFS maps onto these evidence-based interventions in ways that might allow us to offer treatment approaches more accessible for some of our clients. It begins by discussing types of exposure-based treatments for OCD—the only evidence-based psychotherapeutic interventions that have been demonstrated by research to have an impact on OCD. It concludes with a series of case studies showing the benefits and limitations of these exposure-based treatments, continuing to lay the groundwork for Parts III and IV of this book, which show how IFS for OCD complements empirically supported interventions.

Exposure as the Mechanism of Healing

While clinical evidence for the efficacy of exposure-based interventions is impressive, our understanding of the mechanisms and principles underlying that efficacy is still evolving. What we do know is that their success lies in the fact that exposure-based therapies, including traditional ERP, are highly experiential. It's seldom helpful to talk to clients about their OCD or explain logically to them that their estimations of threat are excessive. First, they usually know it, and yet they still experience fear. Second, if an explanation does seem plausible, it has the potential to become a new compulsive strategy. For example, if a therapist says, "Your anxiety response to this situation is excessive. You are actually safe," a client may take this statement and repeat it over and over: "My therapist said I'm safe and my fears are excessive. My therapist said I'm safe and my fears are excessive. My therapist said I'm safe and my fears are excessive." And so, the "intervention" inadvertently becomes part of the disorder.

However, exposure *exercises*, through direct experience, can help clients realize that their original threat appraisals were inaccurate. For instance, clients who have found it frightening to touch everyday objects such as doorknobs and have felt the need to engage in some ritual to alleviate that fear can learn otherwise by successfully taking the risk of touching the objects; in these instances, they find that the fear itself is no longer dangerous because they have felt it and survived. Through exposure to a feared experience and the prevention of a ritual in response, clients find that their fear diminishes over time, and eventually their symptoms diminish as well.

Therapists who use ERP therapy with our clients generally begin with psychoeducation to bring the key feature of response prevention into focus. We explain that a well-balanced nervous system is designed to detect threats, alert a person's entire brain–body system, and then return to a state of calm. In OCD, however, obsessions stir up threat detection and alerts *and then* compulsions short-circuit the cycle's natural ability to balance and settle. This interruption prevents the learning that would typically reinforce a friendly acceptance of a nervous system doing its job in a balanced way. Once this interference causes the system to go too far off track, natural rediscovery of that balance is impeded. From the IFS perspective, parts performing compulsions are highly efficient up front but take over too quickly. To alter this increasingly powerful hijacking of behaviors, we need to offer the client a new experience. We will discuss this more in Part IV, but this aspect of psychoeducation alone can be greatly unburdening for many.

ERP therapy has two parts. First is the "exposure" piece, which intentionally brings the triggering stimuli to the forefront, causing the client to experience the obsessions that arise: uncomfortable thoughts, feelings, images, urges, and sensations. Then, the "response" (or "ritual") prevention piece encourages the client to choose *not* to engage in the corresponding compulsions. The efficacy of ERP has been explained by two main psychological mechanisms: habituation and inhibitory learning.

The Habituation Explanation

The initial theoretical foundation for therapy was not clearly articulated and demonstrated until psychologists Foa and Kozak (1986) presented their emotional processing theory (EPT) in a seminal paper still widely read today. EPT posits that by asking a client to repeatedly confront a triggering stimulus while refraining from engaging in compulsive behaviors, an "unlearning" will occur. According to EPT, *habituation* (i.e., a decrease in fear due to repeated exposure to the feared stimulus) represents new learning, causing a *fear structure* to be replaced by a "non-fear structure." EPT posits that by offering clients a new experience—coming into contact with the feared stimulus, activating the fear structure, and *not* engaging in the escape behavior—clinicians can, through repetition, facilitate several newly learned corrective lessons. One of the most important is that the "fight, flight, or freeze" response will subside on its own without the client performing the compulsion. Habituation allows clients to incorporate this new information into their experiences of fear while providing the implicit understanding that anxiety is not dangerous in and of itself.

According to EPT, exposures must meet two conditions to be effective. First, they must activate the fear. Second, they must provide a new experience in which the feared consequence is either absent or has been disproven. When utilizing an EPT theoretical model, therapists first explain to the client the need for repeated and prolonged exposure, which continues in sessions until habituation occurs. Together the therapist and client develop a *hierarchy of fears* in which the client's specific triggers are rated from 0 to 10. A rating of 0 represents no discomfort and no urge to fix the anxiety, a 5 represents a strong urge to fix, and a 10 represents excruciating, maximum discomfort and an intense urge to eliminate the threat.

EPT posits that ERP therapy offers a new learning experience by triggering the threat response during the exposure and allowing the system to settle on its own without the compulsive behavior interfering (i.e., response prevention). Therapy is essentially an experiment designed to prove the theory that a natural cycle can occur: After a threat, the system will return to calm. In ERP, the therapist designs ways to test and demonstrate the client's ability to return to calm, beginning with moderately fearful triggers and proceeding up a graduated hierarchy of increasingly challenging exercises. Clients are asked to rate their subjective units of distress before and after each exposure, gathering data for two important factors of ERP therapy: the extent of the habituation during the exposure and the extent to which the habituation holds between exposures. Once habituation successfully occurs at a low level, the therapist and client move higher on the scale, systematically teaching the client there's no need to perform a compulsion to return to a calm state.

However, although habituation is expected to eventually bring calm, this is not always the case. Some people do not habituate easily, and some more sensory-based forms of distress and disgust are less responsive to habituation during exposure. Also, other studies show that successful habituation in treatment doesn't always predict good outcomes in life (Craske et al., 2008). For some clients, an exclusive focus on habituation can become an impediment to emotional growth, improvement in overall well-being, or symptom reduction—especially for the many whose nervous systems don't settle easily. Clients often experience a return of symptoms or renewed fear of the same stimulus in different contexts. Sometimes the original fear is merely replaced with an apparently unrelated fear. The fact that fears may return after a period of time, during stressful events, or in new situations suggests that extinction or elimination of the fear structure may not have occurred. And clients who are willing to undergo the discomfort of exposure therapy for its promise of enduring relief often lose faith when they don't get that relief, a common struggle between a client and an EPT-driven ERP therapist. People don't seem to "unlearn" behaviors, they just learn new ones, and this is the central insight of inhibitory learning.

The Inhibitory Learning Theory Explanation

Research by psychologist Michelle Craske et al. (2008) provides an alternate explanation for the ERP learning process by means of inhibitory learning theory (ILT), which distinguishes between *danger learning* (fear acquisition) and *safety learning* in which a person learns through experience that a situation is not dangerous. Unlike EPT, ILT argues that a client's fears are not eliminated or unlearned over the course of treatment. Rather, these fears are durable, resilient, tenacious about protecting us, and highly resistant to change. Nor do they need reinforcement in order to persist even when, as in OCD, the fears are not rational or realistic.

Instead of attempting to extinguish fear responses, the ILT focus turns to helping clients acquire new safety-based associations with the feared stimuli. These associations then inhibit access to the old fear structure (Craske et al., 2014; Abramowitz & Jacoby, 2016); hence, *inhibitory learning*. This model shifts focus away from the reduction of fear levels during exposure exercises. In this view, a person's danger detection system does not go away; instead, confidence in a more accurate safety detection system grows, and through experiential learning new implicit memory structures develop to "inhibit" the danger system.

ILT as a basis for exposure therapy seems more compatible with IFS. The concept of inhibitory learning is compatible with the idea that we don't get rid of our troublesome parts, but rather develop the internal harmony and confidence to relate to them differently. Inhibitory learning posits that facing the feared stimulus, and all of the learning that goes with that experience, allows a more durable set of new associations and expectations to develop. When people learn that the experience they predicted wasn't as bad as what actually occurred (called *expectancy violation*), they acquire the confidence and self-efficacy to let go of avoidance behaviors. As a result, even though reduction of fear is not the focus of the treatment, fear levels generally diminish over time. With repetition of the experience, safety systems learn and gain in strength, overtaking the danger detection systems and beginning to inhibit them. Protective parts learn through experience that they can trust the Self.

Research on inhibitory learning has shown that safety learning tends to be more contextually bound than fear learning and needs to be practiced. While it sometimes takes only one experience to acquire a fear, it may take many trials to counteract it: Just because the client experiences fear reduction in one situation doesn't mean that experience will automatically generalize to all situations; generalization has to be practiced and sought out—especially when Self-leadership has not been emphasized or accounted for. As a result, ILT therapy has developed new and different protocols for ERP treatment. Although the strategy is still to use exposure to the trigger and prevent the compulsive behavior, the goal is to optimize inhibitory learning so that the new learning is more durable. One of these enhancements focuses on maximizing the discrepancy between the client's expectation of fear and the new learning that occurs during the exposure (i.e., "What did you think was going to happen? What actually happened?"). The larger the gap between what was expected and what happened, the more powerful the learning. Another shift in the delivery of ERP from an ILT perspective is the wider incorporation of a variety of triggers, experiential contexts, and outcomes because they're necessary for the new learning to actively generalize across contexts.

The inhibitory learning approach to ERP decreases the focus on habituation and a focus on a hierarchy of fears; instead, it focuses on areas in which the client feels the most motivation and willingness to change, and it frames the experience of treatment very differently. Before an exposure, clients articulate (1) what they expect to experience, (2) their prediction of the probability that the expected experience will occur, and (3) their perceived ability to tolerate the experience. Afterward, they reflect on the actual experience, rate it, and help their parts to register the update. The therapist helps clients reflect on the discrepancy between what they expected and what they actually experienced as a basis for learning new associations that will inhibit the old ones. Arranging for practice during the client's daily routines creates a situation in which various aspects of the client's real-life setting will act as retrieval cues for the learned inhibitory associations. Exposures include a wide range of experiences, with clients encouraged to evaluate and synthesize what they learn and take note of their developing confidence and increased trust in Self.

The one standard and critical feature of treating OCD is the cessation, or at least initially a pause, in the performance of problematic rituals, safety behaviors, and mental compulsions, which block access to new learning and instead reinforce old learning. Encouraging clients to forgo compulsive behaviors offers them a new opportunity to develop a deeper sense of security and trust in Self. The goal is for danger detection systems to recede or be contextualized so these signals relax into the background, and safety learning can grow in strength, allowing uncomfortable feelings to be a part of life. Arguably, there are many ways to accomplish this goal. The more skillful we can become at providing the demeanor, language, and level of support a particular client needs, the more effective we will be as clinicians and the more impact we will have on OCD.

Experience as the Umbrella Concept

Decades of research and practice show that ERP treatment for OCD, especially when paired with medication interventions, is highly effective for those who complete a course of therapy. Yet there are still some stumbling blocks to success. First, not everyone is able to access a specialist in ERP for OCD. Exposure-based treatments are not commonly taught in most graduate programs, so OCD specialists have had to seek out their own post-degree training in ERP theory and practice. Second, because ERP treatment can be very challenging, not every individual, given the opportunity, is willing and able to fully participate. Indeed, the grim and exaggerated specter of ERP therapists making clients lick toilet seats is still stuck in the popular imagination, dissuading some sufferers from even trying the intervention. Third, even for those clients who do agree to participate, some present significant treatment complications including co-occurring disorders and subtle, or not-so-subtle, compliance issues.

Fortunately, by better understanding why ERP is effective, other approaches that have been embraced clinically over the last 15 years utilize the concept of exposure in more accessible ways while still offering the experiential elements so crucial for people with OCD. Validated exposure approaches for OCD include acceptance and commitment therapy (ACT) and the addition of mindfulness and self-compassion to exposure therapy. These variations on traditional ERP offer additional ways for clients to *be with* the many layers of experience that they encounter during challenging experiences and exposures: thoughts, feelings, sensations, urges, and images. In addition, mindfulness and compassion-focused therapies have demonstrated value for many individuals with OCD and provide a conceptual bridge to some of the highly valuable contributions available with IFS.

Acceptance and Commitment Therapy

ACT is an empirically based psychotherapy that combines acceptance and mindfulness techniques with an exposure approach. While ACT is considered an exposure-based treatment, it differs from traditional ERP in an important way. In ERP, the primary focus is on *doing* the exposure exercises; in ACT, there is more of a focus on *how you bring yourself to* the exposure exercises, which brings it a step closer to the approach practiced with IFS for OCD. ERP says what matters is *that* the client is in contact with the stimulus, while ACT says no: It's *how* you're in contact with the stimulus that matters. Much research and the combined experience of many OCD specialists will tell you that if clients simply try to "power through" the exposures, their effectiveness is decreased. ACT emphasizes the importance of generating psychological flexibility by fostering willingness to commit to valued actions. While clients of ACT therapy still acknowledge unpleasant thoughts/feelings, their motivation is enhanced in the context of personally identified values, such as the need to be with friends and family.

The adoption of ACT in the treatment of OCD addressed many issues for the OCD population, including (but not limited to) willingness and motivation. Therapists who use ACT work with clients to help them turn toward the feared stimulus with curiosity and openness to learning. ACT brings together fundamental and commonly understood clinical processes in a manner designed to help clients increase psychological flexibility and the freedom to respond to life directly. Each of six core processes (Hayes et al., 2006) plays a specific part in the dismantling of the obsessive-compulsive cycle. Fostering *acceptance* undermines the compulsive tendency to try to avoid or control life situations that may have uncomfortable or negative emotional impacts. *Defusion* (undermining attachment to, or fusion with, the content of thoughts and feelings) helps disconnect the obsessive association between an event—actual or internal—and one's experience of it. Experiencing the distinction between the *self-as-context* as opposed to being identified with concepts of self, or the content of thoughts, creates a perspective that helps the client feel safer. *Contacting the present moment*, or mindfulness, brings a person into the actuality of life and out of imagined threats that evoke fear. *Values* provide the motivation and the "why" for *committed action*, which is aligned with those values—bringing all six core processes together in a meaningful way.

ACT brought mindfulness into the exposure framework, adding a dimension to treatment that had been missing and extending the reach of OCD treatment to many who had not been helped by ERP alone. By encouraging a mindful perspective, ACT offers tools for relating differently to emotions, not just evoking and enduring them as in the original conceptions of ERP. Also, rather than attempting to change the content of thoughts, ACT helps to create distance from the literal content of thinking. By fostering present-centered, open, and receptive awareness, ACT helps a person embrace the concepts of leaning into uncomfortable experiences rather than judging and avoiding them: "In a mindfulness context, the past is not analyzed, but rather its expressions in the present moment are compassionately acknowledged and accepted" (Arch & Craske, 2009). Many of these concepts map onto processes in IFS.

Mindfulness and Self-Compassion–Based Exposure Therapy

Whereas exposure treatment focuses on *doing* the change, and ACT expands that to *living* the change through acceptance and committed action in the context of mindfulness, cognitive and behavioral therapies grounded directly *in* mindfulness take the shift a little further, cultivating an approach that is more like *being* the change.

Research suggests that integrating mindfulness and self-compassion practices with ERP can significantly enhance treatment outcomes for individuals with OCD (Didonna et al., 2019). Mindfulness techniques complement ERP by helping clients develop a more accepting and observant relationship with their intrusive thoughts, rather than becoming entangled in attempts to suppress or neutralize them (Key et al., 2017). By learning to observe their thoughts with curiosity and non-judgment, clients can more effectively distinguish between the content of obsessive thoughts and their relationship with these thoughts, reducing their perceived threat level (Külz et al., 2014). Self-compassion practices further strengthen this therapeutic process by providing emotional support during the inherently difficult work of ERP. Many individuals with OCD experience intense shame and self-criticism about their symptoms, which can interfere with treatment engagement and progress. By cultivating self-compassion, patients learn to respond to their struggles with kindness rather than harsh judgment, making them more resilient when facing challenging exposures (Leeuwerik et al., 2020). This self-compassionate stance helps reduce the secondary anxiety and depression that often accompany OCD, creating a more sustainable foundation for recovery. The combination of mindfulness and self-compassion also helps patients develop greater psychological flexibility, allowing them to stay present with discomfort without automatically resorting to compulsions (Strauss et al., 2018). This enhanced tolerance for uncertainty and distress directly supports the core goals of ERP by making it easier for individuals to resist compulsive behaviors while building confidence in their ability to handle anxiety-provoking situations. The curiosity and nonjudgmental, compassionate stance found to be so helpful in these approaches are the core process of IFS therapy.

Inference-Based Cognitive Behavioral Therapy

Newer on the scene, but recognized by the IOCDF as a second-line treatment for people with OCD is *inference-based cognitive behavioral therapy* (I-CBT) developed by O'Conner and colleagues at the University of Montreal in the early 2000s (Aardema et al., 2017). Unlike traditional CBT approaches that focus primarily on challenging the probability of feared outcomes, I-CBT emphasizes the cognitive more than the behavioral aspects of CBT, targeting the obsessional doubt which precedes anxiety. Individuals with OCD often make what O'Connor and Aardema (2013) term a "faulty inference"—drawing conclusions based on imagined possibilities rather than direct sensory information from the present moment. This process, known as inferential confusion, leads individuals to doubt their immediate reality in favor of remote possibilities, even when these possibilities contradict available sensory evidence. For example, a person with contamination OCD might look at their visibly clean hands and still conclude they are contaminated based on an elaborate chain of "what if" scenarios, effectively dismissing their direct sensory experience in favor of imagined possibilities. While not an exposure model, I-CBT is experiential, and it does not preclude exposure but utilizes it in conjunction or as a follow-up when appropriate.

The client engaging in I-CBT learns to identify and diminish doubt by paying close attention to present-time sensory data, ultimately using these skills to adjust the story that OCD is telling. Following a structured progression that O'Connor et al. (2005) outlined in their clinical manual, the therapist first helps the client identify their dominant doubt sequence and the underlying inferential confusion. Then, through various exercises, clients learn to recognize when they are abandoning their senses in favor of imagined possibilities, distinguish between reality-based and imagination-based doubts, develop trust in their direct sensory experience, and challenge the reasoning process that leads to doubt, rather than just the content of the thoughts.

I-CBT progresses through 12 modules, a process much too extensive to cover here. However, several key concepts are important in relation to IFS. The first is *inferential confusion* and the reasoning process that sets up *obsessional doubt*; that doubt sparks a sequence of maladaptive reasoning that ends in an *obsessional story*. The focus in I-CBT is on addressing this *obsessional sequence* itself so that crippling anxiety doesn't arise, and exposure becomes unnecessary. IFS for OCD would attribute such maladaptive reasoning processes to the activity of managers, who exist in order to preclude any possibility of actualizing the feared possible self (*FPS*).

Second, I-CBT highlights the fact that the source of the obsessional story can be found in the FPS: that is, the core fear or dreaded future identity or state of being that the person with OCD fears they could become or might secretly be. The FPS is not the truth about the person: It represents the opposite of the person's actual core values and character and is defined by the qualities the person most abhors. Obsessional themes (*subtypes*) develop around the FPS, also known as the Vulnerable Self Theme (O'Connor & Aardema, 2013). In IFS terms, the FPS is not a part. Rather, it represents the burdens (negative beliefs and stuck feelings) carried by the exile. I-CBT identifies some common qualities of an FPS; it is careless, negligent, unlucky, immoral, unlovable, harmful, or insufficient. These qualities and others are also familiar burdens identified in IFS.

A third key concept of I-CBT is the difference between reasonable doubts and obsessional doubts, teaching clients to learn how to trust their five senses, their common sense, and internal sense data (O'Connor et al., 2005). Therapists help clients notice their selective use of out-of-context facts, drawing on technically true but irrelevant information to support their obsessional doubts. Someone might focus on the fact that bacteria can survive on surfaces for days, while ignoring the context that most environmental bacteria are harmless, for instance. This process of beginning to notice the source of the doubt, which IFS would attribute to unblending and becoming more Self-led, allows clients to see OCD as imaginary: a part with a misguided but positive intention.

Next, we explore the concepts of the *OCD Bubble* and reality sensing. Clients learn that their obsessional states of mind are characterized by a high degree of absorption in their frightening, imaginary world: The OCD Bubble. Conversely, they tend to pay a lower level of attention to sensory information from the outer world—the place where they get their data when OCD isn't running the show. By first noticing the Bubble, then choosing to accept the reality of the senses (*reality sensing*) instead, clients are empowered to intervene when they feel pulled toward the imaginary world. Reminding clients of the positive attributes that define them in areas of their lives that are *not* impacted by OCD helps to anchor these clients in a felt awareness that differentiates true Self from obsessional narratives. From an IFS perspective, the exile lives in another place and time: a non-reality that is comparable to the OCD Bubble. Reality sensing fosters a shift in attention and a return to what I-CBT calls the *Real Self*, which in IFS equates to accessing the Self.

Finally, by helping clients dismantle the way the OCD story is constructed and believed during OCD-triggered situations, and by helping them to return to trusting their senses and their sense of Self—in all areas of life—I-CBT helps prevent relapses. Addressing the root thinking patterns that generate OCD symptoms, clients learn to identify their tendency toward inferential confusion so that they're better equipped to catch and correct these thinking patterns before they spiral into full OCD episodes. Similarly, IFS promotes a capacity to detect parts when they begin to take over, solidifying Self-leadership as the more predominant mode of functioning.

In both I-CBT and IFS, we are helping clients directly experience what Self feels like, so that they can more quickly catch and stop OCD in its tracks. Rather than requiring exposure and habituation, both I-CBT and IFS help clients develop the awareness that their doubt can be ameliorated by Self-awareness so, eventually, the FPS (i.e., the burden) has been released and the debilitating anxiety is not triggered.

When Evidence-Based Treatment Falls Short

To demonstrate how I might utilize the methods described in this chapter, I continue the case studies of Justin, Aracelli, and Scott. In later chapters, I return to these cases to show how IFS for OCD can pick up in places where evidence-based therapy has plateaued or hit a roadblock.

Successes and Roadblocks with Justin

When I first met Justin, he had been in a decade or more of talk therapy that did not address his OCD at all—which had grown steadily worse over time. After an initial assessment of Contamination OCD, and building a hierarchy of fears as a reference point, we began his therapy with ERP to help him make some quick improvements and regain the hope that his OCD could get better. We started where Justin was most willing to work, allowing his motivation to dictate what came next so that we could help him acquire new safety-based associations with a feared stimulus of his choosing.

Justin was highly motivated to become more comfortable petting his dog. This was an ideal place to begin: Even though petting his dog offered a low level of threat with a moderate urge to remediate, he had avoided doing it anyway "just in case." Justin made progress and moved on to more challenging exposures until he got to the items toward the top of his hierarchy of fears: encountering chemicals like pesticides and gasoline or using a public toilet without performing his extensive rituals. At this point, he became unwilling to keep going. He tried but found that he couldn't resist the urge to first avoid contamination and then to wash excessively. Having hit a wall in his treatment, he decided he'd rather just limit his life and keep doing his compulsions than face these fears without engaging in elaborate rituals that could take hours every day.

We had now reached an end of the efficacy of traditional exposure treatments for Justin's OCD. At this point, we discussed integrating IFS. Since I am always working from an IFS perspective, he was familiar with parts language and was willing to do anything that might help him—anything other than using ERP to face his fears head on. In the interest of helping Justin find the freedom to live the life he wanted, we shifted to an IFS-informed approach to address his remaining struggles.

Successes and Roadblocks with Aracelli

Aracelli suffered primarily from Harm-focused OCD with some features of Perfectionism. The OCD inventories that Aracelli completed ranked the fears she wanted to address by difficulty and by importance in her life. She decided to start ERP with low-level items related to driving because these obsessions had the greatest impact on her family's routines and she wanted to get comfortable driving the kids to school.

Aracelli was initially able to move through various items along her hierarchy of fears, experiencing inhibitory learning and expectancy violation, thereby causing her to realize that facing fears wasn't as bad as she anticipated and to learn that her feared outcomes would not occur.

Exposure approaches, both ERP and ACT, fell short for Aracelli because of the deep shame she felt when intrusive images would pop into her head. A critical voice told her it would be her fault if something happened to one of her family members and she had done nothing to prevent it. A shift into IFS offered a way for her to befriend and heal the parts who had experienced trauma in her own childhood, so she could return to making choices from a Self-led state.

Successes and Roadblocks with Scott

Scott suffered primarily from moral scrupulosity and other intrusive bad thoughts. When we began ERP, Scott wanted to start with his superstitious rituals such as tapping and knocking on wood to prevent bad things from happening. These improved quickly with ERP. With these successes behind him, Scott wanted to address the issue most troubling to him: his obsession with moral scrupulosity, which was damaging his grades as well as his social life. But Scott's fears of not accurately representing himself and being a "liar" proved more difficult to address using exposure. Scott found he was having a lot of obsessions, and try as he might, he couldn't stop reassuring himself compulsively. This set the stage to begin integrating IFS, to help him be with the insecurities in a relational way instead of just tolerating them.

Refining Current Approaches and Integrating IFS

As the field of OCD treatment evolves in an attempt to meet the needs of individuals with OCD, a shift has occurred away from an exclusive focus on symptom reduction, understanding that one of the limitations of the habituation model of ERP is that the clinician's and client's focus on anxiety reduction can actually get in the way of progress. An emphasis on expectancy violation and maximizing learning has led to more personalized exposures and recognition of the importance of cognitions during exposures. In addition, clinicians who have treated many individuals with OCD, and who have seen the damage OCD can do to a person's work life and relationships, have learned that symptom reduction is only the beginning of the help and healing that many of these clients need.

As our understanding of how exposure works has become more nuanced and sophisticated over time, it seems reasonable to take note of wider applications of the principles of exposure. What if, as Jeff Szymanski, the former executive director of the International OCD Foundation suggested in his preface to this book, by *exposure* we simply mean that we help clients orient toward an experience they previously avoided with an attitude of openness and the willingness to experiencing something new? When we turn *toward* something feared, we change our relationship with it, and we may learn something new about it that we had never noticed before. Turning toward has the power to shift one's experience, to *befriend* it—a key principle in IFS.

The concept of loving your enemies is as old as the hills, a prevalent theme that runs through ancient literature and spiritual traditions. It has persisted because it is also very practical. With respect to OCD, this fundamental attitude of "face it and embrace it" is essential, but too often that gets reduced to a "face it, then drop it" approach. The embrace really matters. The more fully and willingly a person participates in this existential *encounter*, the deeper the transformation. Many people benefit from adopting the stance that they are fighting OCD, even when they must brace themselves to get through the fear. But those who do an about-face and instead open themselves to the very fears that OCD tried to avoid, and do so with curiosity and courage, have a different experience. I have seen IFS make this type of engagement possible for clients who might not have been willing or able to face it otherwise.

Knowing that OCD is as varied and complex as the individuals who have it, our intention is always to keep the client in mind. Rather than simply applying familiar techniques and expecting the client to "get over" any "resistance" to those techniques, we can bring our curiosity and compassion to bear by adapting our language to the needs of the client. If we can do that, feeling secure in the knowledge that our approach is sound and effectively addressing the debilitating condition that we are treating, then why would we not want to offer an approach to the therapy that best suits the client in front of us?

References

Aardema, F., O'Connor, K. P., Delorme, M., & Audet, J. (2017). The inference-based approach (IBA) to the treatment of obsessive–compulsive disorder: An open trial across symptom subtypes and treatment-resistant cases. *Clinical Psychology & Psychotherapy*, 24(2), 289–301. https://doi.org/10.1002/cpp.2024

Abramowitz, J. S. (1998). Does cognitive-behavioral therapy cure obsessive-compulsive disorder? A meta-analytic evaluation of clinical significance. *Behavior Therapy*, 29(2), 339–355. https://doi.org/10.1016/S0005-7894(98)80012-9

Abramowitz, J. S., & Jacoby, R. J. (2016). *Obsessive-compulsive and related disorders: A guide for clinicians*. Oxford University Press.

Arch, J. J., & Craske, M. G. (2009). First-line treatment: A critical appraisal of cognitive behavioral therapy developments and alternatives. *Psychiatric Clinics of North America*, 32(3), 525–547. https://doi.org/10.1016/j.psc.2009.05.001

Craske, M. G., Kircanski, K., Zelikowsky, M., Mystkowski, J., Chowdhury, N., & Baker, A. (2008). Optimizing inhibitory learning during exposure therapy. *Behaviour Research and Therapy*, 46(1), 5–27. https://doi.org/10.1016/j.brat.2007.10.003

Craske, M. G., Treanor, M., Conway, C. C., Zbozinek, T., & Vervliet, B. (2014). Maximizing exposure therapy: An inhibitory learning approach. *Behaviour Research and Therapy*, *58*, 10–23. https://doi.org/10.1016/j.brat.2014.04.006

Didonna, F., Lanfredi, M., Xodo, E., Ferrari, C., Rossi, R., & Pedrini, L. (2019). Mindfulness-based cognitive therapy for obsessive-compulsive disorder: A pilot study. *Journal of Psychiatric Practice*, *25*(2), 156–170. https://doi.org/10.1097/PRA.0000000000000368

Foa, E. B., & Kozak, M. J. (1986). Emotional processing of fear: Exposure to corrective information. *Psychological Bulletin*, *99*(1), 20–35. https://doi.org/10.1037/0033-2909.99.1.20

Foa, E. B., Yadin, E., & Lichner, T. K. (2012). *Exposure and response (ritual) prevention for obsessive-compulsive disorder: Therapist guide* (2nd ed.). Oxford University Press.

Hayes, S. C., Luoma, J. B., Bond, F. W., Masuda, A., & Lillis, J. (2006). Acceptance and commitment therapy: Model, processes and outcomes. *Behaviour Research and Therapy*, *44*(1), 1–25. https://doi.org/10.1016/j.brat.2005.06.006

Key, B. L., Rowa, K., Bieling, P., McCabe, R., & Pawluk, E. J. (2017). Mindfulness-based cognitive therapy as an augmentation treatment for obsessive-compulsive disorder. *Clinical Psychology & Psychotherapy*, *24*(5), 1109–1120. https://doi.org/10.1002/cpp.2076

Külz, A. K., Landmann, S., Cludius, B., Hottenrott, B., Rose, N., Heidenreich, T., Hertenstein, E., Voderholzer, U., & Moritz, S. (2014). Mindfulness-based cognitive therapy in obsessive-compulsive disorder: Protocol of a randomized controlled trial. *BMC Psychiatry*, *14*(1), 314. https://doi.org/10.1186/s12888-014-0314-8

Leeuwerik, T., Cavanagh, K., & Strauss, C. (2020). The association of self-compassion with obsessive-compulsive disorder severity and cognitions. *Journal of Obsessive-Compulsive and Related Disorders*, *27*, 100562.

McKay, D., Sookman, D., Neziroglu, F., Wilhelm, S., Stein, D. J., Kyrios, M., Matthews, K., & Veale, D. (2015). Efficacy of cognitive-behavioral therapy for obsessive–compulsive disorder. *Psychiatry Research*, *227*(1), 104–113. https://doi.org/10.1016/j.psychres.2015.02.004

Meyer, V. (1966). Modification of expectations in cases with obsessional rituals. *Behaviour Research and Therapy*, *4*(4), 273–280. https://doi.org/10.1016/0005-7967(66)90023-4

O'Connor, K., & Aardema, F. (2013). *Clinician's handbook for obsessive-compulsive disorder: Inference-based therapy*. Wiley-Blackwell.

O'Connor, K., Aardema, F., & Pélissier, M. C. (2005). *Beyond reasonable doubt: Reasoning processes in obsessive-compulsive disorder and related disorders*. Wiley.

Strauss, C., Lea, L., Hayward, M., Forrester, E., Leeuwerik, T., Jones, A. M., & Rosten, C. (2018). Mindfulness-based exposure and response prevention for obsessive compulsive disorder: Findings from a pilot randomised controlled trial. *Journal of Anxiety Disorders*, *57*, 39–47.

Part III

The Theory of IFS for OCD

Chapter 6
An IFS Conceptualization of OCD

As described in Part I of this book, Internal Family Systems (IFS) therapy is a clinically developed modality that eschews *talking about* issues in favor of a more direct and experiential healing experience. As described in Part II, obsessive-compulsive disorder (OCD) is a serious condition that is usually best treated with a cognitive behavioral approach, which requires specific training and experience on the part of the therapist. Because of the nature of the processes at play in the development and maintenance of OCD, I believe that IFS theory and practice can be a valuable supplement to empirically supported treatment, or a beneficial way to facilitate it, especially since the effective mechanisms of those methods are consistent with the principles of the IFS approach, as I demonstrate in Chapter 8. However, integrating the IFS model with OCD treatment must be done carefully and conscientiously in the interest of not perpetuating the potential problem of people spending years in treatment that's ineffective. It makes sense ethically to use IFS primarily when treatment via evidence-based models has been only marginally successful or when—for whatever reasons—a client chooses not to, or cannot, engage in these approaches.

The chapters of Part III of this book introduce the theory of IFS for OCD, providing the underpinnings for its rationale and methodology, beginning here in Chapter 6 with a theoretical conceptualization of OCD through the lens, and in the language, of IFS theory. Chapter 7 explains the cyclical nature of the perpetuating dynamics in OCD, from both the conventional and IFS perspectives. Chapter 8 lays the foundation for Part IV by outlining the effective processes of the practice of IFS for OCD, and how its techniques map onto empirically supported methods for OCD treatment.

This chapter begins by answering the question of why practitioners might consider using IFS to help treat OCD. It continues with an explanation of the terminology of IFS for OCD and then presents an IFS-informed description of the fundamentals of OCD, viewed as the interactions among protective parts engaged in an obsessive and compulsive behavioral loop attempting to eliminate distress and uncertainty.

DOI: 10.4324/9781003449812-10

Why IFS for OCD?

At first glance, IFS therapy may seem incompatible with traditional therapies for OCD. On the one hand, cognitive behavioral therapy (CBT) with exposure and response prevention (ERP) guides clients through manualized steps designed to help them face feared situations and gradually change their cognitions and behaviors with the intention that these changes will eventually reduce their levels of symptom-provoking anxiety and distress. In contrast, IFS therapy does not target cognitive or behavioral change; instead, it aims to heal underlying core issues, with the intention that the experience of healing releases the constraints of negative beliefs and burdens, thus reducing symptomatic behavior.

But several aspects of IFS therapy make it particularly valuable in OCD treatment. First, it focuses on facilitating clients' access to their sense of Self and helps them relate differently, *from* Self, to the parts of them that engage in problematic patterns. Starting with Self as the primary agent in clients' recovery, rather than, for instance, relying on a hierarchy of fears as a measure of success, helps regulate the pace of therapy and ensures that clients' willingness is real and not merely performed by an aspirational or compliant part wanting to make progress. Demonstrating trust in clients' wisdom can help therapists avoid typical treatment derailment that can happen when therapy moves too fast or when clients inadvertently undo treatment gains by engaging in safety-seeking behaviors or compulsions, during or after therapy, due to backlash from parts who were not on board with the treatment plan.

Second, although IFS therapy takes place in deep conversation between a therapist and a client, it is not talk therapy in the usual exploratory sense. Rather, the therapist facilitates an internal process that is inherently *experiential*. IFS therapists help clients to get to know parts of themselves that have strong feelings or disturbing thoughts by fostering some differentiation and by encouraging some curiosity and ultimately openness and compassion. The underlying principle is that IFS therapists guide clients to turn toward internal experiences (thoughts, feelings, sensations, images, and urges) that they would otherwise avoid and face them with enough perspective to welcome the experiences rather than be overwhelmed by them. Much like cognitive therapy and other mindfulness-informed approaches, IFS also facilitates the recognition that learning *not* to identify with the experience ("I have an anxiety" instead of "I am anxious"), leads clients to discover that they have more options than simply avoiding the thoughts and feelings of their parts or reacting strongly against them in an attempt to eliminate them. In addition, IFS takes the neutral observer stance a step further by bringing attention to the response of the part being acknowledged. It's not just compassion that can initiate a reciprocal relationship with parts: *Any* of the qualities of Self described in the 8 C's—curiosity, confidence, or calm, for instance—can help parts feel the presence of Self and relax.

Third, IFS is *experimental* in that it encourages clients to be scientists, offering options for their parts to try new things. We ask parts to see for themselves how well Self handles a feared experience that the protectors were working hard to manage or extinguish. The focus on healing as a process of discovery involves a method of inquiry that relies upon the moment-to-moment experiences of the client in a session as a guide rather than on therapist-directed change. Clients set not only the sequencing and pace of treatment but also the direction of their growth toward lives that *they* value. This is what IFS calls being experience-near, meaning that we recognize that clients make highly personal associations within the material they bring to therapy, associations arising from individual, life, and cultural experiences. Weaving the highly personal associations and the experimental approach together, IFS can stay very close to the emotionally relevant material without teetering into reinforcing OC processes. This balance allows IFS therapists to treat the whole person without detracting from our ability to address OCD symptoms safely, adding immensely to the impact of therapy without reinforcing obsessions and compulsions. Clients' increased agency has a positive impact on both their motivation and their courage in the face of OCD.

This synthesis of the behavioral mindset of exposure therapy with the relationally attuned IFS model has many benefits. First, it makes recovery possible for people who cannot access or do not experience sufficient relief—for a variety of reasons—through conventional ERP. Second, by bolstering readiness and willingness, it makes it less likely that people will experience backlash or relapse or an unhelpful aversion to ongoing therapy for co-existing issues after ERP. Third, it offers a way to compassionately address OCD in daily life by welcoming the difficulties in valued experiences instead of staying mired in a constant internal battle or need to ignore. Challenges once felt as internally adversarial can become opportunities to learn, befriend, and integrate one's inner world through a freeing engagement with the external one.

The Language of IFS for OCD

Because IFS theory conceptualizes mental disorders as the activities of protective parts that have become extreme, and because I have found that through the lens of IFS, OCD is actually the work of a cluster of parts that have taken on very specific roles within a person's overall system and their neurobiology, I refer to OCD as the *OC subsystem,* and its recurring obsessive-compulsive sequence as the *OC cycle.*

IFS emphasizes that parts are far more than just the roles, behaviors, or burdens that they carry: They have a wide range of feelings and capacities. Nevertheless, we often recognize them by what they do, and so it is natural to initially call them by names that represent their actions. For instance, many people might relate to having an angry part or an avoidant part. In practice, as therapy progresses, IFS therapists have the flexibility to inquire more deeply about the full range of a part, and clients may choose to call the part by a different label, or even a proper name, that more fully suits their own experience of it. Because I am aiming for clarity in this book, I label parts according to their function as obsessional and/or compulsive—without meaning to diminish the complex nature of this internal cast of characters.

It would be efficient here to simply describe all protectors within the OC subsystem as *OC protectors* and I do use the term whenever possible to refer generally to protectors engaged in the OC cycle. However, at times it's important to distinguish between the activities of the two types of OC protectors. The proactive managers in the OC subsystem primarily engage in obsessions, so I call them *obsessional* or *OC managers*. Similarly, the reactive firefighters in the OC subsystem primarily perform compulsions, so I call them *compulsive* or *OC firefighters*. Precision is important here, because the language of OCD, as used colloquially, can be imprecise. As awareness of OCD has grown in society, people often use the word "obsessing" to refer to ruminative thoughts, in which they think things through over and over in an attempt to reduce their distress—a mental activity defined in the OCD community as compulsive. Also, people often mistakenly use the word "obsession" to mean someone or something they are thinking a lot about. For these reasons, I use the word "obsessional" to describe the quality of the OC managerial thought process, which produces doubt, distress, and anxiety.

Finally, when I discuss the theory explaining why IFS works with OCD, I call the approach "IFS for OCD," but, as I explain in Chapter 8, I call the actual process of treatment "Self-led ERP."

What's Different about OCD?

As we saw in Chapter 1, parts represent our personalities, traits, strengths, and weaknesses, and they are how we interact and engage with the world. When these parts fulfill their preferred roles, Self is not only accessible but also orchestrates the effort, producing an internal system that's both balanced and harmonious. Each of an individual's various parts has a voice, and the parts work in harmony under the direction of the Self.

Sometimes, however, "a part can take over mentally and make us see the world through its eyes" (Sweezy, 2023, p. 8). IFS calls this *blending*. It's natural for parts to blend and unblend in mild ways that support functioning. In a highly blended system where Self-leadership is weakened, the threat of worries and pain dominating awareness causes protectors to work harder and use more extreme methods: Controlling managers and disinhibiting firefighters now make enemies of the vulnerable ones who are burdened with negative convictions (*I am . . . bad, alone, inadequate*, and so on). Extreme managers become more critical and exacting, attempting to create peace and predictability by hiding, banishing, or trying to improve vulnerable parts—thereby stirring up even more pain for and from them. Agitated firefighters react in any way they can—often rashly—to that pain once it surfaces in attempts to soothe, numb, or annihilate it. These managers and firefighters generally end up in conflict. The more harshly managers push for achievement and control, the greater the pressure for firefighters to offer relief, often undoing the work of the manager and resulting in an unhappy stalemate. IFS calls this a *polarization*: a relationship in which the work of one protector is at cross purposes with the other (Schwartz & Sweezy, 2020).

However, in a system where OCD has taken hold, obsessional managers and compulsive firefighters form a powerful *alliance* that can obscure and limit access to Self. In traditional OCD parlance, obsessions stir up anxiety and compulsions neutralize or remediate it. Viewing OCD through the lens of IFS, we see that a specific subset of managers and firefighters exhibits increasingly extreme and repetitive behaviors in response to what we might think of as "sticky" fear circuitry in the brain. Together, these OC protectors are engaged in a team effort to ensure that the parts who have been saddled with uncertainty and dread, fearful beliefs, intolerable possibilities, and disturbing feelings are exiled. Believing, from their perspective, that they're contributing to the overall wellbeing of the person, their extreme convictions urge them toward ever more symptomatic and intractable behavior. In this way, the OC managers and firefighters create a subsystem within the overall system, escalating their protective behaviors and manifesting obsessive and compulsive symptoms.

This subsystem becomes identified as OCD.

What's Different about IFS for OCD?

As we adapt IFS therapy to be used with a greater number of clinical issues and diagnoses, we will likely need to make some adjustments to the typical practice of IFS therapy, which posits that the behavior of protectors and exiles is primarily psychologically based and motivated. As shown in Chapter 3, such is not always the case when OCD takes hold. In addition to psychosocial factors, other considerations—genes, viruses, infections, autoimmune disorders, injury, and neurodivergence—can all factor into the development of the disorder.

Incorporating Neurobiological Factors

The "OCD brain" has the problem of reacting disproportionately to stressors ranging from everyday insults to severe traumas—and the mind of the person with an OCD-inclined brain has the extra problem of protective parts incorrectly experiencing vulnerable parts as the source of threatening overstimulation. OCD often involves a lower activation threshold for a brain pathway that creates an alarm system that causes exaggerated concerns about danger, hygiene, and harm. OC protectors attribute each of these concerns to a part and attempt to exile it. The exiles receive the blame and become burdened with uncertainty, confusion, or the belief that they are potentially at fault. Having OCD can be a trauma in and of itself as parts hear these frightening messages and come to believe that they *may* have a harmful identity.

Taking into account the neurological contributions to OCD, IFS therapy understands that the divergent neurobiology of the brain for many people with OCD can put pressure on the internal systems of parts, whose ever-alert protectors respond to biological alarm signals, regardless of their origin and validity, akin to a neuroceptive mismatch in which the clients' internal reaction to a situation is disproportional to the situation itself. The reverse may be true in some cases as well; parts may push the OC button to distract from other concerns. Either way, the overactive brain circuits seen in many people with OCD can cause exiles to continue to experience traumatic wounding in the present as protective parts obsessively make associations that induce and deepen pain or connect present reality with pain from the past or the imagined future. The OC cycle of proactive and reactive protection, effective in the short term, is increasingly damaging in the long term; the brain's alarm system and the mind's OC protectors continue to shame and hurt vulnerable parts, generating even more fear and uncertainty as well-meaning obsessional managers create a backstory to explain the signals of the brain. This explains the traumatic nature of having and living with OCD: Clients may become traumatized, or further traumatized, by their own OC protectors, whose accusations and disturbing content frighten exiles, adding to burdens of uncertainty, shame, and guilt. The client's entire system, OC and not, can become bathed in this shame and guilt, creating other challenges such as depression down the line.

From the perspective of IFS theory, the crux of the issue is twofold: First, protective parts in an OC subsystem take on extreme roles, making *scary meaning* and creating intrusive thoughts to protect the system from being overwhelmed by messages from a sticky brain circuit that is highly sensitive to danger cues. (For the obsessional manager, scary meaning is better than no meaning, which is why its efforts end up being overwhelming.) Second, OC protectors make a cognitive error in trying to restore the balance to the system by attributing the reason for those thoughts to exiles and subsequently neutralizing them. For example, a protector in an OC subsystem may blame and seek to exile a sensitive part for its feelings of guilt, when in fact the concern about having hurt someone is coming from the manager's hypervigilance and storytelling. The conclusions reached by these protective manager parts are not based in reality but are instead a form of confusion. They do not understand that overly sensitive hardwiring in the brain is generating a false alarm. They do not understand that the vulnerable parts, which are alerted when the alarm system goes off, are *the recipients of* a problem rather than the origin of it. They do not understand that their hypervigilance, exaggeration, and persistent conscious attention to these possible threats (contamination, taboo thoughts, asymmetry, potential harm, etc.) further activate the exiles, which only adds to the problems posed by the glitchy brain circuit. These misunderstandings are particularly unfortunate because many exiles may already be confused about the origin of their burdens, wondering *Am I a bad or dangerous person?* As firefighters perform compulsions to neutralize the putative external threats, their actions temporarily soothe the obsessional managers and bring limited relief to the exiled parts. This repetitive, ritualistic behavior does not actually help the exiles, who are now additionally worried by the belief that they're the problem. Over time, the load of confusion, alarm, and shame infuse the entire system, which only serves to fuel the subsystem's OC cycle.

Understanding the OC Cycle

Obsessional managers are always at a heightened state of alertness, vigilantly scanning for triggers—or even the possibility that they might encounter a trigger. Triggers may be external or internal and can result from neurobiological glitches, the burdens of exiles flaring up or from thought–thought fusion, which creates self-fulfilling prophesies. Fears of having the OCD thoughts *create* the OCD thoughts. Bypassing Self, obsessional managers sound alarms, scan for data, and make associations. They tell *what if* stories, elaborating on the possible disastrous consequences and high likelihood of the frightening possibilities they imagine. Vulnerable parts receive the signals and feel threatened. Typically, obsessional managers increase their alarms until firefighters rush in, either to assuage the exile, calm the manager or both. *What ifs* are the hot potato in an OC subsystem. They are the shared concern of OC protectors and exiles, the production of obsessional managers directed at exiles and extinguished by compulsive firefighters. This shifting of blame occurs over and over in an escalating cycle, ultimately undermining the agreed-upon intention of well-being.

Bereft of the moderating influence of Self, compulsive firefighters pounce on oversimplified and misdirected solutions—seeking reassurance, mentally reviewing, washing, checking, etc., with ever more urgency—momentarily restoring a sense of safety. By applying these surface-level solutions to complex and nuanced problems, compulsive firefighters achieve highly effective—but unfortunately short-term—results. Still, these apparent solutions seem to work, which encourages obsessional managers to seek repeated help from the firefighters.

Exiles receive the blame from the team of OC protectors, hearing that they *may be or already are,* in fact, bad, dangerous, inadequate, or vulnerable. The whole system may come to believe that the exiles themselves are at fault. And if exiles in the larger system carry burdens that represent highly personal material, usually involving uncertainty about vulnerabilities or feared possibilities about the Self or identity, OC protectors will latch onto these vulnerabilities, imbue them with scary meaning, and then guard against them at all costs. That is what OC protectors are committed to accomplishing. In order to keep what they see as the exiles' true nature under wraps and out of awareness and minimize the impact of the intolerable burdens they carry, OC protectors create narratives that induce behaviors designed either to prevent or avoid the expression of or contact with the exile or to evoke compulsive rituals to reinstate a sense of safety once the exile has been disturbed.

Self-Leadership and OCD

As discussed in Part I, Self is undamaged and always available to us. The trick is helping our parts clear the way so that we can access it. Sometimes described as a state of consciousness, Self is characterized both by a natural clarity and compassionate awareness and the absence (or reduced intensity) of constraints imposed on us by parts who have agendas of their own. We can't do much about our parts arising with their thoughts, feelings, sensations, images, and memories—that's what they're supposed to do—but by being centered in and connected with Self, we are able to orchestrate how we respond to these parts. With Self in the lead, our parts themselves grow calmer, more flexible and confident, and more trusting that they can rely on Self to be there: a *virtuous* cycle. The more we access Self-energy, the easier it becomes.

But what happens when OCD takes hold is that a person's everyday protectors begin to work extraordinarily hard to manage the ongoing biological vulnerability in the brain, accidentally creating obsessive and compulsive thoughts and behaviors that escalate, leaving very little room for Self. People with OCD frequently call these repetitive thoughts *loops* or *spirals*. The stories that OCD tells begin to displace present-moment awareness, replacing sensory data from the real world with hypothetical, anxiety-inducing stories designed to fix imaginary problems that stand in for deeper core fears. The protectors that form an alliance to guard this OC subsystem guide choices and actions to such an extent that Self has no opportunity to demonstrate another perspective and recover leadership. Eventually, a person with OCD lives more and more in an imaginary world of *what ifs*.

In such a world, OC protectors lay claim to an overwhelming amount of power and control. For example, where an ordinary organizing part is helpful in everyday tasks, such as emerging when a person wants to tidy up a room and receding when the task is reasonably done, obsessional organizing parts can make people feel that they *have* to keep their room *perfectly* tidy *or else*. The part *takes over*, leaving no room for Self to decide how much or how little organizing is appropriate. The room gets organized in both cases, but the first situation includes options around timing and extent, and it results in satisfaction, whereas the second is accomplished through rigorous rules that have very little to do with reality and may bring relief only if done to perfection—and then only temporarily. Avoidance of the rigor of such an all or nothing endeavor can result in the room staying messy. Protectors in an OC subsystem seem Self-like at first, which allows them to operate for a while before they're recognized as problematic. This is why an innocuous behavior, such as a tendency to organize, can become highly challenging in a person with OCD.

A person whose Self has the trust of protective parts experiences a sense of internal harmony, spaciousness, awareness, connectedness, and perspective. In a Self-led state, a person is also rooted in consensus reality and common sense. Generally, IFS therapy can help resolve the issues that plague most people by healing exiles so that protectors are willing and able to release polarities, soften, relax, or step back, that is, to recognize and make space for Self and the clear-sighted confidence that comes with Self-leadership. However, the task is more complicated in people with OCD, where the Self's healthy leadership has been hijacked by the neurobiology of a sticky brain circuit, which the person's protective system works frantically trying to manage both by triggering it and responding to it. IFS therapy for OCD goes to the heart of this hijacking and recognizes that we're not just dealing with challenging protectors. While the obsessions of a person with OCD are traditionally thought of as nothing more than arbitrary, involuntary intrusions sparked by the brain, many clinicians are beginning to explore the extent to which a person has agency to intervene in ways that soften the impact of these intrusions and their ability to activate anxiety and distress. Through its attention to increasing access to Self, IFS for OCD offers a way to amplify the agency inherent in every person, fostering awareness of Self, and rebuilding all parts' ability to know and trust that Self is both present and capable of being the system's guiding force.

When OC Parts Take Over for Self

Clients with OCD often say, "What if ... ?," "I have to ... ," and "I can't ..."—expressing how much they identify with parts that feel compelled or constrained. When IFS therapists hear these statements, we know that we aren't hearing Self; we're hearing parts posing as Self. Although this blending with parts happens in clients with any number of concerns, an escalation occurs when the teamwork between obsessional and compulsive protectors gives them so much influence in the overall system that other parts begin to defer to them as if they were Self. Self then becomes almost entirely eclipsed. OC protectors who have taken over leadership assume urgent responsibility for instilling security in the person's psychological system—both from perceived external threats and from the impact of burdens carried by exiles. This is why they often act in an intimidating and self-righteous manner. Not only are they convinced they are right, but they are also often convinced they are the Self.

IFS theory sees psychological issues and symptoms as the work of increasingly extreme protective parts working hard to keep exiles out of awareness. We see a system that is no longer balanced and harmonious but instead disconnected and often out of touch with a sense of Self. In IFS therapy for OCD, the patterned dynamics between parts become warped and magnified: We see OC protectors taking safety-seeking to such an extreme that their work becomes highly destructive. We see OC protectors working together not only to provide a reasonable sense of safety and security but—the unique OCD burden—also to eliminate uncertainty and eradicate the possibility of distress altogether. Extreme in the name of safety, completion, balance, and certainty, OC protectors are difficult to tone down.

Obsessional Managers Stir Up Alarm and Doubt

Whereas the managers of any internal system are tasked with the overarching job of protecting it by planning ahead, taking care of basic survival needs, and promoting growth and progress, obsessional managers have the added burden of responding to a glitchy brain. Managers are all concerned about preventing emotional pain, and so they are socially attuned and aware of consequences. When they become obsessional they may take these same activities to the extreme, imagining potential danger, insensitivity, or slights and becoming increasingly insecure and unable to accept the normal ambiguities of life. Making unrealistic inferences of danger or imagined transgressions, they seem to be responding to both the OC brain's low threshold for sending alerts and its greater difficulty getting to resolution. Obsessional managers routinely engage in thought patterns that align with what Foa et al. (2012) described as the primary cognitive errors of obsessions. They (1) assume in advance that any alert signals a high probability of actual danger, (2) exaggerate the cost of the danger to get the attention of firefighters, and (3) require constant and complete proof that there is absolutely no risk of danger in the current moment. These tendencies make obsessional managers the tough customers they are known to be. They get triggered very easily (often by prompts invisible to other people), and they have a harder time feeling complete or satisfied. Doubt continues to plague them long after other managers might be assuaged or persuaded to relax.

As the sentries on the lookout for any suggestion of a threatening vulnerability, obsessional managers manufacture stories about exactly what they are attempting to avoid. They intend to prevent feared consequences from occurring, but their repetitive presentation of frightening or disturbing thoughts, images, and concerns generates increased focus on the distressing content. They prefer to keep a person terrified of a catastrophic outcome, no matter how unlikely, rather than risk it possibly occurring. These obsessional managers are highly dedicated to their mission and become increasingly determined to keep a person safe at all costs. They often feel that they are not working hard enough, even though they are exhausted, and they have a tough time believing that if they relaxed, the result would not be catastrophic.

The tone of these obsessional managers can range from mildly alert to frantic as they engage in a wide variety of strategies to keep the system alerted to potential risks. They may scan for feelings, urges, and sensations to the extent that they keep a person up all night searching for fearful contents to latch onto. They may worry about the possibility of having a scary thought thus creating the scary thought. Their intention or job is to prevent the possibility of something bad happening, even at the cost of sounding false alarms and stirring up anxious, guilty, and shameful states.

Obsessional managers also have characteristic *methods* that distinguish them. Because they presume a high probability of danger and a high cost as a result of the imagined dangerous events, this catastrophizing drives them to act like Chicken Little, announcing dire predictions, threatening other parts, blaming, and judging any failure to pay attention. Requiring absolute proof that the presumed danger will not happen drives them to recruit firefighters to remediate contamination, be scrupulously certain, perfect, or "just right." They have learned that amplifying their noise—becoming very loud, demanding, and intimidating or shaky and concerned—is the most effective way to alleviate their doubt.

Common obsessional parts that take over for the Self include noticers, scanners, assessors, evaluators, trackers, threateners, blamers, helicopter parts, hypervigilant parts, warning parts, *what if* and *uh-oh* parts, as well as all manner of control panel monitors, switchboard operators, and security guards. Some of them focus on sensations such as tingling fingers or genitals, others send visuals such as gruesome images or disturbing scenes. These obsessional parts stir up the system with triggering content, and amplify the alerts until they get a response. As the self-appointed keepers of this sticky brain circuit these protectors believe they are responsible for interpreting its signals, hitting panic buttons, and recruiting responders.

Compulsive Firefighters Remediate and Neutralize Fear and Doubt

As the emergency response team within the internal system, compulsive firefighters shoulder many responsibilities and often take them to the extreme. To do that, they frequently attempt to repair imagined or hypothetical damage that, if true, would confirm the OC subsystem's greatest fears. Compulsive firefighters have infinite strategies to calm exiles and assure the managers that they have eliminated all possible threats. Physical and mental rituals, safety behaviors, and reassurances can be tailored to the individual with great precision. While some compulsions—such as checking, planning, or being perfectionistic—with the intention of preventing anxiety may seem like proactive managerial parts, they can also function as compulsive firefighter reactions to the fear of having anxiety or distress.

Whereas obsessional managers are motivated into action by the possibility of their worst fears coming true, compulsive firefighters are usually motivated by the exhortations of obsessional managers and the feelings of the exile they stir up. They believe it is their job to alleviate any sense of danger—real or imagined—no matter what it takes, even if the remedy is unpleasant, repetitive, and difficult. As part of this responsibility, compulsive firefighters perform as many safety behaviors as necessary to momentarily pacify frantic managers and calm the fearful exiles. Pretty quickly, the OC protectors and many other parts notice and learn that certain rituals are effective in alleviating distress. And because of the sticky brain circuit that repetitively intrudes with obsessions, they are called on to perform these rituals over and over again. Initial one-off safety behaviors become compulsory, then automatic. Losing sight of what is best for the system as a whole, compulsive firefighters become relentless and severe, bypassing and obscuring Self with their tunnel vision approach to safe-keeping. Creating an illusory structure of safety and certainty comes at the cost of knowing and trusting Self, as well as the ability to live a free and courageous life. Together, obsessional managers and compulsive firefighters attempt not only to provide a reasonable sense of safety and security but also to eliminate all uncertainty and eradicate the mere possibility of distress.

Exiles in OCD Carry Themes and Burdens of Uncertainty

Although specific OCD themes fall loosely into the standard umbrella categories of subtypes of OCD discussed in Chapter 4, their content is highly personal. The specific details that OC managers become drawn to are related to, but are often a distraction from, or a cartoon-like, extreme caricature of the fears of vulnerable parts that have been exiled. In short, although not representative of the true nature of the Self, the themes of obsessions are also not entirely random (Aardema et al., 2005). Inference-base CBT (I-CBT) posits that obsessions tend to be organized around a Vulnerable Self Theme (O'Connor & Aardema, 2013), which in the IFS model would correspond to the negative beliefs or burdens of exiles. Like I-CBT, IFS connects the themes of OCD to a "feared possible self"—an untrue, negative belief about the self. The feared negative belief or anticipated possibility becomes the focus of the obsessions, and this connection determines the type or theme of OCD. Although not the cause or the perpetuating factor in OCD, the very personal themes when framed as the burdens of exiles can inform treatment as we will see in Chapter 11.

Exiles are not bad parts but vulnerable ones who received a bad message or experienced something bad. The remnants of that message, the beliefs they took on about themselves, represent the opposite of who a person truly is and wants to be. For instance, a person who values being conscientious, considerate, and kind may have protective parts that guard against thoughts, feelings, or fears about potentially being or becoming careless, irresponsible, selfish, aggressive, or violent. The increasingly extreme protective efforts made to keep these parts exiled blocks access to and even awareness of Self.

The Feared Possible Self can dictate the theme of the OCD, but there is no one-to-one correlation between the theme of OCD and the nature of the exiles that the OC protectors are guarding against. There are, however, some common patterns that I have noticed. Contamination-focused obsessions recruit de-contamination compulsions to quiet down or exile parts carrying shameful, stuck feelings of being dirty or disgusting, vulnerable to illness, permeable to unsavory qualities, or fearful of being overtaken by states believed to be intolerable. Harm and responsibility-focused obsessions aim to protect the individual from feelings of guilt, of being at fault, or of being a bad, careless, or irresponsible person. These exiles may come to fear being fundamentally to blame for having caused harm or being a bad person. In another example, violence and sexuality-focused obsessions aim to protect the individual from possibly being or becoming dangerous, evil, perverse, or bad. These obsessional narratives weave stories of horrifying possibilities that scare and shame exiles, who may come to believe that their nature makes them not just unlovable, but actually harmful to others. Symmetry and rightness-focused obsessions intend to protect the individual from feelings of being incomplete, wrong, off, or imperfect. These exiles develop burdens and beliefs related to not being good enough, of failure, of not fitting in, and of feeling wrong or off. They often stir up feelings, pressure, and irritation that manifest as agitation. Religion and morality-focused obsessional managers aspire to ensure that individuals have not veered from the loftiest goals of their religious strictures or strayed from high moral standards. Imperfection in these areas creates shame, fears of being outcast, impostor fears, and guilt.

The experiences of exiles are highly varied and idiosyncratic whether they are inherited, arise from personal experience, or are developed in response to protector alarms. In all of these cases, while lived experience may have made an exile vulnerable to the burdens that inform an OC theme, any personal burdens from that lived experience are spotlighted and exacerbated by the OC protector activity: They are not the cause or the driving force of it.

Protectors' Burdens Fuel the OCD System

IFS theory draws a clear distinction between the inherent traits, capacities, thoughts, and feelings of parts and the burdensome beliefs and traumatic feelings they have become stuck with. The burdens of exiles are the focus of the healing steps of typical IFS treatment because they are the reason that most protectors become extreme in the first place. OC subsystems, however, generally do not develop out of—and so are not driven by—a perceived need to eliminate exiles who carry personal burdens from traumatic experiences. *Any* part can have a burden, and OCD is typically more perpetuated by burdened protectors, who are likely to create or magnify the burdens of exiles by sounding incessant and disturbing alarms that frighten vulnerable parts of the system. Exiles may be primed to receive these messages from obsessional managers who seem to pick on their vulnerabilities to get their alarm message across to the compulsive firefighters. Helping burdened protectors let go of this need to alarm the system is a particular focus in IFS for OCD and will be discussed in Part IV.

To fully grasp and recognize the subsystem of parts that present as OCD, it is helpful to note that OC protectors often carry an overwhelming sense of responsibility for dealing with the perception of threat, instability, and danger. Though it is a job at which they can never fully succeed, they typcially believe that they are the only ones who know how to keep the system safe. From their perspective, protectors in OCD can never rest, as they are defined by their never-ending and repetitive jobs.

Obsessional managers proudly believe it is their responsibility to handle all aspects of the alarms, many of which are rooted in faulty brain circuitry. They do this by a combination of vigilance and making up backstories to create an explanation for the danger signals and a rationale for continuing to sound alarms. Protector burdens may be inherited and are frequently held onto and even prized. The obsessional narratives they create are frightening stories often developed to explain unconscious neural processes or neuroception (Porges, 2007). Our nervous system evaluates environmental cues for safety, danger, or life threat without conscious awareness; parts commonly respond to and push these biological buttons. These alerts or signals pass by unannounced for most. But for someone with OCD what might otherwise be a benign flare from the nervous system becomes what I have been calling a brain glitch. This perception of fear is interpreted by the obsessional manager, who tries to make meaning of the signal and then directs it at vulnerable parts. In the process OC managers may blame or even terrorize vulnerable parts viewed as or accused of being dangerous. The obsessional stories created by OC managers often start with "what if. . ." or "could it be. . ." and they are designed to ensure safety by getting the attention of the whole system. The unfortunate result is increased confusion, fear, or shame on the part of an exile. Exiles may develop burdens of guilt or pain from the experience of being sacrificed or scapegoated for the sake of the protective agenda by OC protectors who team up to create the illusion of safety and control by first stirring up an obsessional alarm and then neutralizing it with a compulsion.

This IFS approach to OCD allows clients to connect with all these parts and to come to know them more intimately, creating many more opportunities to intervene. Viewed through this lens, exiles can be recognized as casualties of the obsessional managers' crusade to create cognitive backfill to support their false alarms; firefighters are the parts they recruit to determine with absolute certainty that their doubts and fears are not actualized or already true. The very OC processes that provide some relief reinforce the association of the exile with the trigger and reinforce the likelihood that protective parts will continue to exert massive amounts of energy to get rid of the parts they have blamed: the exiles.

References

Aardema, F., O'Connor, K. P., Emmelkamp, P. M. G., Marchand, A., & Todorov, C. (2005). Inferential confusion in obsessive–compulsive disorder: The inferential confusion questionnaire. *Behaviour Research and Therapy*, 43(3), 293–308. https://doi.org/10.1016/j.brat.2004.02.003

Foa, E. B., Yadin, E., & Lichner, T. K. (2012). *Exposure and response (ritual) prevention for obsessive-compulsive disorder: Therapist guide* (2nd ed.). Oxford University Press.

O'Connor, K., & Aardema, F. (2013). *Clinician's handbook for obsessive-compulsive disorder: Inference-based therapy*. Wiley-Blackwell.

Porges, S. W. (2007). The polyvagal perspective. *Biological Psychology, 74*(2), 116–143. https://doi.org/10.1016/j.biopsycho.2006.06.009

Schwartz, R. C., & Sweezy, M. (2020). *Internal family systems therapy* (2nd ed.). The Guilford Press.

Sweezy, M. (2023). *Internal family systems therapy for shame and guilt*. The Guilford Press.

Chapter 7

The OCD Cycle through an IFS Lens

Understanding OCD in the language of Internal Family Systems (IFS) involves both defining the component parts and how they interact as a system. Chapter 6 described obsession and compulsions as protective parts that either stir up anxiety and distress (obsessions) or work to neutralize and remediate it (compulsions). It explored core fears based in themes held by vulnerable parts that have been exiled. But in addition to the parts involved in psychological multiplicity, the other guiding principle of IFS is that these parts relate internally as a system—much like a family system. Intervening with one member inevitably impacts the whole. In this chapter, we will look more closely at the obsessive-compulsive (OC) cycle and elaborate on the dynamic, non-linear relationships among the obsessional managers, compulsive firefighters, neurobiology, and the other parts within the larger system.

This IFS for OCD framing of the OC subsystem has two particularly distinctive features. The first, as explained in Chapter 6, is that, unlike more typical internal conflicts that manifest as polarizations, OC protectors tend to show up as an alliance between obsessional managers and compulsive firefighters. The OC manager–firefighter alliance creates a powerful dynamic with the intention to eliminate any possibility of relevant threat to the person. Obsessional managers amplify the intensity of their alerts until they convince compulsive firefighters to jump in with rituals or other safety behaviors. Ironically, this teamwork creates greater fear and uncertainty, leading to increased dependency on the OC protective agenda.

The second distinctive feature is that IFS for OCD sees this as a *dynamic and relational* cycle, which means it can start at any point, and the signals—the hot potato—can move in many directions. The standard description of the OCD cycle begins with a trigger and proceeds through obsession to distress to compulsion and then relief—in a straight sequence. Although obsessions usually kick-start the cycle, clients report that an OCD spiral can begin at any point and proceed in a variety of ways. From a systems perspective, we know that an intervention with any part of the cycle

DOI: 10.4324/9781003449812-11

will affect the whole and, consequently, each part of the whole. Knowing this allows us to be more attentive to the needs of the client and their parts, whether the ones who show up first are (1) the *uh-oh* representing first awareness of the brain signal, (2) the obsessional manager's interpretation of this neurologically generated *uh-oh* as dangerous, (3) a compulsive firefighter neutralizing the fear with rituals or mental rituals, or (4) an exile surfacing with challenging feelings that fuel OC protectors. Any of these may be presumed to occur in response to an external or internal trigger. External OCD triggers, which can include an item, a person, or an occurrence—for instance, a social media post or a classroom assignment—may be perceived and responded to by any part. Internal OCD triggers, likewise, might prompt action from any part, and these include thoughts about having a thought (thought–thought fusion), thoughts perceived as dangerous, or a bodily sensation. Understanding the cycle as a dynamic system, IFS for OCD allows us to intervene in a fluid and flexible manner at any point in the cycle and to concurrently address non-OCD parts that may be fueling the OC subsystem. In this way, we can have an impact at both the level of precipitating and the perpetuating factors of OCD. This will be discussed further in Chapter 8.

This chapter describes the interactions between system-wide non-OCD parts and those within the OC subsystem. It begins by discussing what OCD feels like to the sufferer, then presents the dynamics of the OC cycle in more detail. It continues with an explanation of how the OC cycle takes over, then describes some of the ways the parts in the OC subsystem interact with the larger internal system.

What OCD Feels Like

Imagine that a person with Harm OCD feels a bump in the road while driving. Although the driver can see a large pothole in the rearview mirror, that's not reassuring. An obsessional manager whose job it is to scout for danger initiates a doubting sequence, firing off a flare in the form of an intrusive, reflexive *uh-oh!* Motivated by uncertainty—the worst possible truth for OC subsystems—the obsessional manager puts the OC subsystem on high alert and a team of obsessional parts (an alarmist, a storyteller, etc.) begins to work proactively to stir up enough anxiety that the person will take action to make 100% certain that everything is actually OK. This process may stir up an exile who struggles with a burden of shame about possibly being a bad person, or a vulnerable part may accept blame. By the time the cycle has happened a number of times, the vulnerable exile is primed to feel guilt and/or shame. Ostensibly to calm the exiles that they have just intentionally stirred up, the OC protectors need the person to compulsively check, perform a reassuring compulsive ritual, or engage in some other safety behavior. "What if that was a person in the road?" the obsessional manager worries. "Is it possible that I hit someone?"

At this point, some reasonable part, a rational or critical manager, for instance, may try to dismiss the intrusions and alarms—"Don't listen to the OCD, we have things to do—that's ridiculous! You know you don't need to worry about that"—to no avail. As alarmist and storytelling managers escalate, the OC subsystem drowns out the dissenting parts, making a case for the possibility that the bad thing actually *may* have happened and enumerating all of the potential consequences if it did. If reasonable parts still argue, the obsessional managers up the ante and start shouting character assassinations: "A person may be lying there dying, and if they die, it'll be your fault." "What kind of person wouldn't at least check?" These comments continue to get to the sensitive exile, who feels even more shamed and overwhelmed, and answering the increasingly loud alarm, the compulsive firefighters spring into action: "Go back!" they plead. "We have to check the road!"

The issue that the obsessing manager wants to focus on is the possible hit-and-run rather than the insecurity of the exile struggling with its burden: the fear of possibly being a bad person or the belief that it's already true. But both the trigger and the exile are there alongside the sticky brain circuit commanding attention and increasing the agitation of the OC manager. So, the obsessional manager continues to make a case for doubting what happened on the road until a firefighter becomes willing to bring the driver back to the intersection to check, proving that the driver is a virtuous and caring person, and did not harm anyone. When that has been accomplished, the obsessional manager and exile are momentarily relieved and settle down. But because there is a sticky brain circuit, the obsessional protectors get triggered again by another *uh-oh*: "Maybe the person was thrown into a ditch," the driver thinks, with a sinking feeling. "Maybe they crawled to the side of the road, and I didn't see them when I went back." These thoughts and feelings are as subjectively real as having actually seen a person dead in the road—and the OCD process continues.

Over time, people with OCD experience a rapidly increasing disconnection from the inner wisdom of the Self as OCD damages their ability to trust their capacity to look at real data in real time, and to make sensible choices based on reality. They begin instead to identify with the OC protective system and join it in its effort to keep dread, distress, and uncertainty out of awareness. Clients with OCD often say that they no longer know whether something is safe. They don't trust themselves. They don't know who they are without their obsessions and compulsions, and they certainly don't know what to do or not do. They are worn out from the exhaustion of living with the cumulative stress of an OC subsystem that baits their whole system stirring up alarm, confusion, and shame. They believe they are flying blind, but Self is there: They just don't know it.

106 Internal Family Systems Therapy for OCD

The Dynamics of the OC Cycle

As explained in Chapter 3, researchers of OCD represent the conventional OCD cycle as a circular process. The cycle starts with a trigger, leading to an obsession that causes distress, which then prompts a compulsion, resulting in temporary relief that reinforces the likelihood that the cycle will continue. See Figure 7.1.

But IFS allows us to see a person's actual experience of OCD as much more dynamic without making it complex. Through the lens of IFS, the OC cycle appears as a subsystem of *interactions* among proactive obsessional managers, who stir up the whole system with doubt ("What if. . .?"); reactive firefighters, who attempt to fix the concerns; and the unhappy exiles who are the parts left holding the distress. Obsessional managers can function like switchboard operators or command central; responsible for collecting and processing data, getting the message out to parts that need to act and dialing up or down the level of intensity. They can speak to exiles, compulsive firefighters, and any other parts willing to listen. For these reasons, I find the OC subsystem may best be captured through an adaptation of the IFS triangle introduced by Cece Sykes (2017, p. 30) in her discussion of addiction. Her model puts managers and firefighters at the top of an inverted triangle and shows their positions as a polarization that attempts to keep the exile at the bottom of the diagram out of awareness. My adaptation understands the OC subsystem as a conversation among teams of

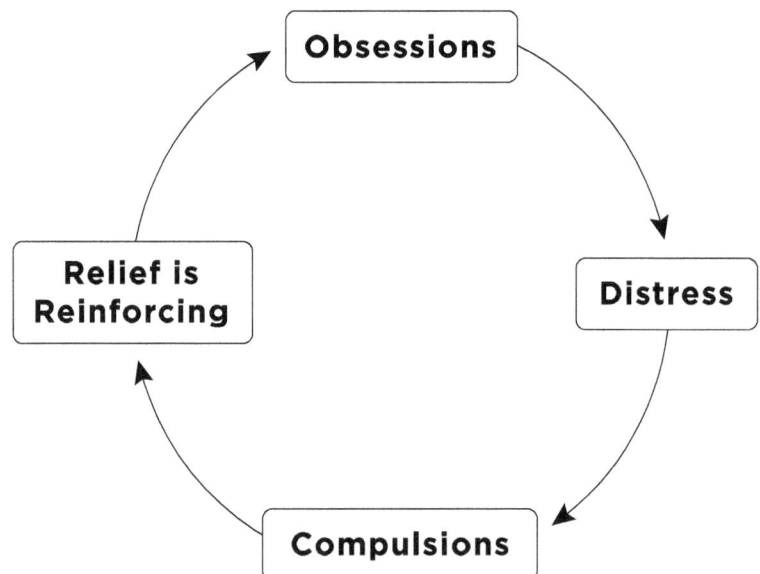

Figure 7.1 The OCD cycle.

obsessional managers and teams of compulsive firefighters. It also places the uncertain and otherwise burdened exiles they protect at the bottom. I call this diagram the *dynamic OC cycle* (see Figure 7.2).

This diagram shows the many ways that multiple internal conversations occur and circulate among managers, firefighters, and exiles. Exiles, parts that are pushed out because they carry feelings of distress, uncertainty, and vulnerability, are the focus of protectors. But it is useful to point out that the trigger can stir up an obsessional manager, an exile, or both. Throughout the cycle, as this chapter will show, the conversation can go in multiple directions. Sometimes there are multiple OC subsystems that focus on different fears. Although this sounds complicated, the one primary goal of IFS, developing Self-leadership, remains the same, and helping one part will always help the whole system.

Consider Scott, who had both a scrupulosity subsystem and a contamination subsystem. He would approach the writing of an essay in the mindset of his morally scrupulous manager who relentlessly worried about whether he was representing his topic accurately. An exile would be stirred up and pour shame and dread into the system, which the compulsive firefighter of his scrupulosity subsystem would soothe by checking his essay yet again, *just to be sure*. At the same time, his contamination manager would seek to explain his nameless dread by hyper-focusing on what he was touching and creating a story about his computer keyboard being dirty. This contamination-focused OC manager could be organized around the same exile, or a different one (who feared dying) than the scrupulosity-focused manager (who felt he might be bad or guilty). This new warning, via an obsessional narrative about being contaminated, would get Scott's firefighters to do

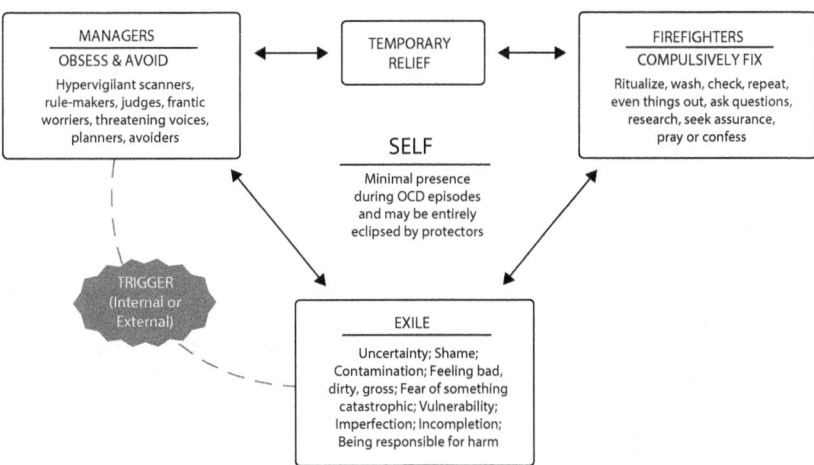

Figure 7.2 The dynamic OC cycle.

rituals, which took him away from writing his essay, causing other parts, including hyperachievers, to get riled up. Scott would leave his desk to clean his phone and wash his hands, then, upon returning to the essay, his scrupulosity manager would once again urge him to start over to make sure that he had not plagiarized, and the whole process would repeat itself.

How the Dynamic OC Cycle Takes Over

OC loops usually begin when something triggers an intrusive obsession. An obsessional manager receives these inadequately filtered signals, creates a story about what it might mean—usually blames or frightens a vulnerable part—and then recruits firefighters to banish the part when it gets stirred up. The trigger can activate the person's whole OC protective subsystem, showing up in a wide array of possible forms, including alarming thoughts, detailed images of what could happen, uncomfortable sensations of contamination, feelings of dread, and/or unwanted urges. Obsessional managers such as vigilant parts and scanners look for support to corroborate the possibility that the obsession is pointing to danger and must be acted upon. They shout threats and focus on the uncomfortable sensations, while their assessing partners begin using this data to weave tales of catastrophe—generally combining it with irrelevant associations, hearsay, and imaginary consequences to generate elaborate hypotheticals.

The game plan of these managers is to prevent catastrophic threats: either imagined proximal danger, such as *I will get sick and die,* or abstract dangerous possibilities, such as *I will lose my mind* or *I will feel like this forever.* They do so by shifting awareness to obsessions that can be relieved by compulsions. However, instead of preventing catastrophe or anxiety about catastrophe, these proactive protector parts cause more distress, doubt, shame, dread, physical pressure, or agitation by stirring up the person's core fears, which are held by the exiles.

In a non-OC system, exiles are certain they are unlovable or bad as a result of experiences that they themselves have had at a time in the past when the burden was created. In OC subsystems, while exiles may have had such experiences, that's not always the case. Often, they carry confusing burdens of uncertainty and fear that are a result of the intensity caused by intrusive thoughts. These intrusions cause managers to anxiously predict dire outcomes and firefighters to perform extreme behaviors to ensure certainty and safety. Thus, exiles swim in a distinctive pool of OCD-generated fear and anxiety, wondering if they are the cause of the intrusive thought and its potential dire outcomes.

As the obsessional managers double down on alarm bells about what "might" happen, firefighters jump in to use compulsive behaviors to neutralize, rationalize, fix, undo, or otherwise get rid of these vulnerable states of uncertainty, fear, or shame. Because firefighters tend to be very effective at offering short-term relief, their voices grow in intensity. "Managers, don't worry about those *what-ifs*—I fixed them." The obsessional managers and compulsive firefighters congratulate each other, agreeing that the problem has been solved. Unfortunately, none of the OC protectors addressed the actual problem: the absence of a clear connection to the compassion and courage of Self. Because OC subsystem relief has been brokered by protectors rather than Self, it builds no trust in Self because no risk or challenge has been taken. Self has had no opportunity to demonstrate how its calm presence and perspective can manage doubts and uncertainties. And so, obsessional managers are validated for their alarm, compulsive firefighters are rewarded for their efforts, and the OC loop is reinforced.

Because the overarching goal of all IFS therapy is to reestablish a healthy relationship between parts and Self, our standard intervention is to suggest to overactive protector parts that a better way to help the system restore balance is to unburden exiles and return responsibility to Self. But because the OC cycle reflects an internal system in which protectors are dealing with glitchy neurobiology, the standard intervention is often not enough. This is where OCD-informed IFS therapy can have a significant impact. Protectors have pushed Self way into the background because they don't understand that only Self can contextualize these neurobiologically triggered obsessions. Even though obsessional managers may initially relax once the chronic uncertainty represented by an exile is resolved by the IFS healing steps, the brain with OCD may continue to send intrusive thoughts. The sense of relief will be brief, and the obsessional managers will feel the need to jump back in to re-exile the vulnerable parts that had been retrieved . . . and the cycle begins anew.

Protector Interactions

In the external world of family dynamics, when one family member begins to behave differently, others notice and adapt. The same is true with internal family systems: our individual parts live and interact in dynamic internal relationships that evolve and affect each other as they change. And—not surprisingly—the more moderate parts of many people with OC subsystems grow increasingly frustrated by, or even feel terrorized by, the OC parts.

OC subsystems have their own OC relationships, *and* they live within the complicated alliances, hierarchies, polarities, and polarizations of a person's overall internal system. Aligned against the larger system, OC parts stand in unison as other parts polarize with the OC subsystem. In other words, non-OC parts have their own agendas regarding the subsystem that has come to be known as OCD. These reactions can be beneficial when balanced and compassionate, and lead toward treatment that is effective; or they can be less productive, when their distractions become destructive or addictive or their judgments evoke shame. This struggle greatly affects how OCD progresses over time, how people engage in and respond to therapy, and how people feel about themselves in relation to their OCD. Protectors that polarize with OC protectors can create shame about having OCD, exacerbate the OCD, and prevent a person from seeking or engaging in treatment—this is why we will address them first in Part IV.

Alliances within the OC Subsystem

As explained in Chapter 2, parts sometimes work together because they have compatible skill sets. For instance, organizer parts may work with people pleasers to make sure things get done on time. These alliances are particularly strong in OCD because it takes teamwork to try to be absolutely certain all the time. In OCD, managers recruit firefighters and work with them rather than against them in an attempt to eliminate all doubt about their concerns. There is a functional relationship between obsessive and compulsive parts in OC subsystems: Obsessions stir up anxiety and compulsions relieve it. In IFS language, obsessional managers join forces with compulsive firefighters, recruiting them to maintain the perceived safety of the subsystem. Firefighters either see themselves as *partnering* with obsessive managers to exile the parts with distressing feelings or as needing to calm down both the exile and the managers. The managers are perpetually on the lookout, scanning for danger, making associations, sounding alarms, warning, taunting, shouting rules, and threatening that they will not stop inciting fear until the firefighters jump in and do something to fix the uncomfortable situation: to clean a surface or hands, to make sure the bad thought isn't true, or to eliminate the possibility of connections between contaminated and uncontaminated things or thoughts.

Exiles in an OC subsystem often report that the obsessions of the manager parts scare them, and many managers acknowledge that that's their goal: They want everyone to be on high alert in order to prevent something really bad from happening. If they can keep the subsystem stirred up enough, they can induce the firefighters to take care of business. OCD firefighters' rituals do work in a very real and powerful way: They have the immediate effect of relieving distress. Exiles, however, usually have deeper concerns that are not being addressed and need a connection with Self to be healed.

Polarizations with the Outer System

Because OC protectors team up to create such a strong and sometimes destructive pattern, they often get into conflicts with other protectors outside of the OC subsystem. There are numerous ways this can happen, depending on a client's overall capacities, proclivities, issues, and traits. For instance, a health-conscious manager may get very upset by an OC decontamination firefighter who—in the name of staying healthy—damages health by wiping until the person bleeds or by using bleach in excess to clean the house. A firefighter with similar good intentions may try to prevent the suffering of OCD by drowning the whole OC subsystem in alcohol or other addictions. Because it's important to identify and disentangle these polarizations, let's look at some common dynamics.

Obsessional managers are burdened by the belief that they are responsible for managing the brain's alarm system and the body's whole nervous system. When the overwhelmed and increasingly burdened manager in an OC subsystem eagerly recruits its corresponding firefighter, urging it to do whatever it takes to fix an identified problem (the scapegoated exile) and bring the subsystem back to equilibrium (even for a short while), it sets in motion a cycle that continues to reinforce itself. OC protectors don't care—and maybe don't even notice—if exiles become collateral damage and further traumatized by their activity. Meanwhile, there are usually some system-wide parts that have something to say about it or engage in a struggle with the OC subsystem as a unit.

Manager–OC Subsystem Polarizations

A person who is sufficiently Self-led has manager parts that interact with the world and conduct the daily affairs of life in an effective, balanced way, consistent with the person's traits and preferred styles. But the focus of *obsessional* managers is primarily on alerting the system to prevent negative states or possibilities. Although their intentions are benign, they act in ways that are not in alignment with the person's own ideas about what's reasonable or understandable. Instead, they react to specific content that serves as a stand-in for core values and concerns and often do it in bizarre and frightening ways.

For example, Justin had an obsessional manager who had extreme concerns and expectations about hygiene that, if engaged in, could take up to three hours to execute. That created conflict with a hyperachieving—although not obsessive—manager part who had lofty goals for his social life and career and who would team up with a critical—also not obsessive—protector who also wanted him to excel and have a social life, and who would berate him for being pathetic, a failure, and a mess. As a result, he would stand for hours debating whether to do his hygiene rituals. A non-compulsive firefighter would then jump in and put him to sleep, thus letting him avoid the conflict. The way forward is to help the non-obsessive hyperachiever and critic give us space so Justin can get to know the obsessional manager's concerns, putting this part in touch with Self who can then make a reasonable call.

Non-obsessional managers, especially high-achieving, treatment-focused managers who are trying to improve the person, tend to get very frustrated with compulsive parts as well. For instance, the high-achieving manager will make the demand that a person not waste time with rituals, either to get something done or for the sake of overly ambitious therapy goals. They might say, "No ritual, we'll never get better if we keep doing that," and the compulsive firefighter will either double its efforts next time or redirect them to a different domain. A critical manager may join the hyperachieving one saying things like "You're ruining my life, OCD!" The compulsive part will make a case for doing the ritual anyway, and with increasing urgency, minimizing the impact of its actions. It might say, "It's so much more expedient. It's no big deal. Just one more time. It's not that bad. It will help."

For Scott, after a compulsive firefighter spends an hour reading and re-reading his paper before submitting it—and then unsubmits it and reads it again to quiet fears that he may have plagiarized—his critical manager would attack saying, "This is pathetic! You know you don't have to read that again. You tried hard enough!" An obsessional manager would reply, "You won't be able to live with yourself!"—and this would spark the whole OC cycle, again. It's hard to polarize with an OC firefighter without an obsessional manager or exile jumping in, because they're the ones who feel that the person is in danger if the firefighter doesn't act. But in this example, the point is that the non-obsessional managers come to hate the actions of compulsive firefighters, just as they can be polarized with any firefighter. And the end result is that the compulsive firefighter doubles down, becoming more extreme.

Firefighter–OC Subsystem Polarizations

Sometimes firefighters, in their role as the parts who douse the pain, make it their job to drown out the complaints of obsessional managers and distract from the anguish caused by compulsions. It's not uncommon for people with strong OC subsystems to have equally strong distractor parts who act out in other ways that are addictive or impulsive. These firefighters, unlike safety- or certainty-seeking compulsive firefighters, will usually say that they are providing relief, anything that feels good or draws attention away from the hypervigilant parts who stir up doubt and the never-ending compulsions.

For instance, Scott is often up all night playing video games, causing his parents to worry about what they are calling a video-game addiction. When queried, Scott's firefighter says that if he stops and tries to go to sleep, the hyperfocusing part will zero in on everything that doesn't feel right or that he could have done wrong during the day.

Since firefighters tend to be highly reactive, they don't care what other problems they may cause. Sometimes, system-wide firefighters who offer distraction or relief can polarize with compulsive firefighters. For instance, addictive processes can become a way to cope with the intense strain and agony of OCD. When a firefighter engages in behaviors such as compulsive gambling, porn or substance use it can directly antagonize the OC subsystem. Concerns about certainty, morality, and safety are exacerbated by the very parts seeking relief. For example, checking compulsions to make sure the stove is off may conflict with another compulsive firefighter, an avoider, who sidesteps the fear of seeing something problematic by staying out of the kitchen.

It can be helpful to note the intention of distractors who are often trying to steer clear of the impact and effects of the OC cycle but their actions are counterproductive. Aracelli, for instance, found that having a few drinks at the end of the day helped her mind to quiet down, but then she found that had more worries that she couldn't be trusted to be sure her kids were taken care of and the compulsions the next day would be excessive.

Hierarchies between Systems

As we've seen, OC subsystems don't exist on their own; they're embedded within larger internal family systems with their own managers and firefighters. When OCD takes hold, obsessional managers and compulsive firefighters team up and can dominate more stable managers and firefighters in internal power struggles. As we have just seen, they can also push other parts into even more extreme roles. As the OC cycle escalates, OC protectors can take over leadership of the larger system, and compel a person to engage in safety-seeking and remediating behaviors that more balanced parts know are unwarranted. This escalation can lead to shame and despair. Many individuals with OCD have fought for years or decades to be able to touch a bathroom faucet or a doorknob without agony. Naming and normalizing the domineering nature of OC parts is essential to help critical, shaming parts soften and allow other parts to feel that compassion is warranted, and courage is possible. Therapists who work with OCD must be able to confidently hold the hope when our clients cannot.

Many people with severe OCD call it a bully; they sometimes say, "My brain makes me do this." One client told me that having OCD feels like your inner system is being "run by the mob": A ritual or compulsion must be performed for the boss, or the whole system will pay a price. Sufferers can experience no rest, no joy, until they do the ritual: They live in what feels like an inner tyranny in which a person's other parts—a manager who wants to feel a sense of accomplishment, for instance—are rendered helpless by a hypervigilant manager who needs to be perfectly sure before making a move.

Through clinical experience with many individuals with OCD who come to see the different features of their OCD as parts, I have found these patterns of alliances and polarizations within and between the system and OC subsystem to be common. While this is by no means the only way to conceptualize OCD in the language of parts, the dynamics described in this chapter—OC protector alliances, and polarizations of the OC parts with other protectors—are very common. As parts become more trusting of Self, they may become able to handle triggers without sparking the OC subsystem into a spiral. We can begin to see parts softening and backing out of their more extreme roles in the OC subsystem and easing into doing jobs aligned with their capacities as parts of the greater whole. For instance, Aracelli did not want a part she began to call her "Bossy Mom" to disappear altogether, but simply to become less bossy and less urgently demanding. Scott did not want to let go of his scrupulous, standard-setting part altogether, but to have it ease into a more reasonable conscientious quality.

OCD is dynamic, complex, and highly idiosyncratic. I believe IFS is uniquely equipped to stay near to and true to the experiences of individual clients without inadvertently reinforcing OCD. By recognizing both the parts involved and how they interact systemically, we can tailor the effective mechanisms of empirically supported OCD treatment to the needs of our clients. In Chapter 8, we will explore how IFS processes map onto some of these therapeutic principles and mechanisms, including exposure, inhibitory learning, mindfulness, acceptance, and emotional processing.

Reference

Sykes, C., (2017). An IFS lens on addiction: Compassion for extreme parts. In M. Sweezy & E. L. Ziskind (Eds.). *Innovations and elaborations in Internal Family Systems therapy* (pp. 29–48). Routledge, Taylor & Francis Group.

Chapter 8

Why and How IFS Can Be Useful for Clients with OCD

Internal Family Systems (IFS) therapists can enhance their ability to treat obsessive-compulsive disorder (OCD) by becoming familiar with effective aspects of traditional treatment, and—where appropriate—by incorporating them into IFS therapy. OCD specialists who use evidence-based approaches can use IFS to help more people engage more deeply in treatment and—in addition to the reduction of OCD symptoms—achieve more stable and long-lasting overall mental health and well being. This integration is an attempt to bring the best of both worlds together in a framework that can be adapted to each individual case as needed.

This chapter provides an overview of how I use an IFS approach for working with OCD and presents the theoretical underpinnings supporting its effectiveness. It proposes a method for using IFS for OCD that I call Self-led exposure and response prevention (Self-led ERP), explaining its basis in empirically validated treatments. This chapter begins by introducing the stages and steps of Self-led ERP, then highlights the main processes at work in each stage and maps these onto the core principles of exposure and response prevention (ERP) therapy, acceptance and commitment therapy (ACT), self-compassion and mindfulness-based therapies, and Inference-based cognitive behavioral therapy (I-CBT). In doing so, this chapter sets the stage for the demonstration of Self-led ERP in Part IV.

An Integrated, Principles-Driven Approach

As we saw in Chapter 2, IFS therapy ordinarily unfolds in two broad phases. The first phase focuses on securing the willingness of protective parts. It uses the 6 F's (Find, Focus On, Flesh Out, Feel Toward, BeFriend, and Identify Fears) to identify and understand the protective parts within a client's internal system, discover who the parts protect, and help the parts unblend from each other and the Self. The second phase focuses on encountering and attending to previously exiled parts progressing through the healing steps (Witnessing, Do Over, Retrieval, Unburdening, Invitation, and Integration) to reintegrate exiled parts and return protective parts to their preferred roles, generally promoting balance and reestablishing Self-leadership within the system.

IFS for OCD differs from standard IFS in two ways. First, we spend more time upfront helping the OC protective subsystem build trust, often suggesting small experiments or exposures encouraging protectors to try something new. Second, after helping the exile or exiles involved, we usually return to those same protectors with greater Self-leadership to help them recognize the shift and to facilitate the generalization of what has been learned on the inside to the world outside. Re-engaging with these protective parts helps them to unburden and to redefine their roles in terms of capacities within a Self-led system.

Self-led ERP is an integration of IFS methods and mind-set with the goals and principles of ERP. This approach is not to be confused with *self-directed ERP*, in which ERP clients are sent home to practice exposures on their own in order to help generalize the learning. In Self-led ERP, we are operating from the premise of multiplicity, in which the psyche operates as a system of parts that represent capacities and traits, as well as patterned reactivity that manifests as symptoms. Reestablishing Self-leadership through intentional encountering of experiences and relating to parts rather than avoiding experiences and exiling these parts is the goal of Self-led ERP.

Because language is important, I want to start this part of the discussion by addressing the terms "exposure" and "response prevention." First, even though my clinical experience has shown me that much of IFS for OCD maps onto standard ERP, the two modalities are not the same. Part of the value of IFS is that it offers a *relational* approach to these processes. I find that the term "encounter" better captures the experience of working with parts and their feelings than "exposure"—which can sound harsh and involuntary. "Encounter" also better describes the quality of simultaneous two-way relationships: The therapist engages with the client and the client's parts, the client's Self engages with their parts, and the client's parts engage with one another.

Similarly, "response prevention" can be a difficult term for some who are concerned it could imply coercion and contribute to a loss of agency. Although that's not the intention, clients with a trauma history can still have a negative reaction. If we instead focus on *relating to protectors* and helping them recognize and trust the Self, they become more willing to step back with some encouragement. This empowers the client and fosters independence. When this kind of encounter happens, no one's parts are controlling other parts or preventing compulsions. Instead, internal Self-to-part relationships cultivate clients' capacity to be with all their parts without being overtaken by protector behaviors. This reframing makes IFS valuable for OCD treatment. When protectors relax, we encounter the exiles and offer to be with them as they reveal their distress. This is the essence of an uplifted and kind ERP within the IFS for OCD framework.

Self-led ERP is similar to standard ERP in that we are facilitating a curious turning toward difficult feelings as opposed to avoiding or attempting to eliminate them, and we are doing that while helping our clients refrain from engaging in compulsive activities. But it differs in two keys ways. First, as mentioned above, what standard ERP calls response prevention is not driven by the agenda of the therapist or the client's managerial parts, but rather by the client's Self. Access to the qualities of Self bolsters the willingness of OC protectors to stand back and allow Self to take the lead. Establishing respectful relationships with protective parts serves the dual purpose of stopping the ritualizing and building internal security, strength, and solidarity. Second, the principle of exposure in ERP is an intentional provocation of distress with the intention to learn that the feelings can be tolerated. Here, when we make contact with distressed parts it is done with compassion, acceptance, and the intention to welcome them back into the system with an open heart rather than fostering a subtle (or not so subtle) wish for them to be extinguished by habituation or simply tolerated. In this approach, ERP can stand for "encounter and relate to parts"—a more IFS-friendly turn of phrase.

We invoke Self-leadership as the guide and invite the client to be the decision maker—as opposed to letting either OCD make the call or dutifully following therapist instructions. We believe that clients *do* know who they are and what is real. Some things are, in fact, certain and they do not need to embrace uncertainty for those.

As a principles-driven approach to addressing this complex disorder, IFS for OCD focuses on underlying mechanisms while remaining flexible in application. The intention is that this approach offers hope to clients across the full spectrum of OCD presentations. As our understanding of OCD continues to develop, the principles-driven approach described by Winston and Seif (2017, 2019) provides a framework that can incorporate new research findings while maintaining focus on the fundamental processes that maintain obsessive-compulsive cycles. We lean upon that approach here with mappings onto additional processes shown to be effective in IFS as well as OCD treatment.

Three Stages of IFS for OCD

Stage One of IFS for OCD begins by helping a client's obsessive and compulsive protective parts pause and recognize Self. Building this awareness of, and connection between, OC protectors and Self creates familiarity, trust, and a greater ability to unblend. This is where we build willingness for "response prevention" by "relating to protectors." We befriend both ordinary protectors and OC protectors, and we are cognizant that the OC managers and firefighters may be louder, more burdened, and more reluctant to step back. Also, we expect to find some important differences in how our negotiations with protectors will go. Interviewing OC protectors about their fears can be agitating and reinforce them, creating more associations and the experience of either sticky thoughts or spiraling. We need to be careful not to engage with the obsessional content or narrative, but instead connect with the part itself, appreciating its helpful intention while recognizing that it no longer needs to function alone. The presence of Self makes the difference.

When both ordinary protectors and OC protectors exhibit an initial willingness to step back, Stage Two begins. We encounter the exile or exiles initially identified by the OC protectors, forging deeper connections with the parts that the OC protectors are guarding. This encounter is the most obvious IFS correlate to exposure. By addressing protector fears up front and as they come back up, we can often facilitate a high-contact—and often surprisingly unguarded—encounter. Clients often report these experiences as being deeper and more intense than they were able to experience in standard ERP. With curiosity and other qualities of Self, clients can stay open to what is arising in the experience, allowing more contact as protectors are learning to trust Self. A part that created a story about why another part needed to be exiled can watch Self contact that exile safely and participate in the experience. We turn toward distressed parts relationally, with compassion, in order to offer witnessing and connection. This shows OC protectors that Self is available to handle exiles' intensity and the larger system can more clearly see the obsessional manager's role in perpetuating the cycle.

Stage Three is an intentional return to OC protectors to update them, help them adjust, and collaborate to rehearse the real-world integration of internal changes. This expansion of the typical two-phase IFS therapy is usually required because of the peculiarities of OCD: While ordinary protectors are generally relieved to let go of their jobs, OC protectors are often not interested and find it difficult to stop doing their jobs even once the OC exiles have been encountered, retrieved, and unburdened. There are at least two reasons for this. First, OC protectors contend with a brain circuit that continues to misfire, and so they will need extra attention and practice in the real world before they are able to fully relax. Second, it generally takes a wider variety of experiences for OC protectors to learn to trust Self and relinquish their extreme roles; obsessional managers continue to monitor and interpret neurobiology and compulsive firefighters also continue to feel at least somewhat compelled to action by the appearance of obsessions and repeated negative reinforcement. This stage can be a time when practicing more traditional experiential exercises or experiments is useful for helping new learning to generalize. These exercises promote relationship building and confidence, and they foster the development of trust in Self among the OC protectors.

The Processes at Work in IFS for OCD

A vast amount of research provides evidence for the effectiveness of ERP as the first-line treatment for OCD. ACT, as an exposure model, is nearly as well established, and I-CBT is also accruing a great deal of evidence to support its efficacy with OCD (although it is still considered a second-line approach). Primarily a clinical model, research on IFS is just beginning. A recent feasibility study found "preliminary evidence for three theoretically relevant mechanisms for PTSD symptom reduction using the IFS-based therapeutic approach" (Comeau et al., 2024). These were identified as decentering, self-compassion, and emotion regulation. The rest of this chapter will look at the processes involved in IFS therapy as we use it with OCD and show how these map onto the mechanisms that we know to be effective in the evidence-based methods for OCD treatment mentioned above. Unique in its ability to approach OCD from both the exposure perspective and to address the roots of OCD in inferential confusion, IFS for OCD both normalizes intrusive thoughts and facilitates disengagement from them. Framing effective principles in the relational language of parts allows for a coherent and cohesive synergy between and among these approaches.

Compatibility of these concepts should make it relatively straightforward for both IFS therapists and OCD therapists to accommodate their own methods within this integrated approach. For OCD specialists, seeing the experiential nature of IFS may facilitate willingness to integrate IFS where it has value, or to use it knowing that the mechanisms at work are the very ones that have been shown to be effective with OCD. For IFS clinicians, it's worthwhile to reinforce the realization that—after centuries of being deemed untreatable—OCD has been found to respond well to a variety of evidence-based methods, so that we can incorporate them in IFS-attuned ways as we work with OC subsystems.

Stage One: Unblending and Befriending

In the early stage of IFS therapy with most clients, "the protectors call the shots." As Martha Sweezy explains, "We ask protectors to unblend; if they decline, we ask why; then we offer to help with their concerns. Eventually, they permit us to help the exiled parts and we move to the second part of therapy" (Sweezy, 2023, p. 115). Much of the time in IFS therapy, healing and unburdening exiles marks a turning point in therapy. With OCD, as mentioned above, it is the protectors who need most of our help.

As in typical IFS, IFS for OCD begins with unblending. Although we continue to facilitate unblending throughout therapy, it is the necessary first move toward unlocking the protective system in service of helping clients access Self-energy.

Whenever parts show up, IFS therapy notes and addresses blending and unblending. With protective parts, this is the initial and sometimes, if they are mild-mannered and cooperative protectors, the only move necessary. With exiles it is just the opening for healing to come. Unblending is the doorway to Self-leadership and all of the C's that come with it. By finding a connected but differentiated perspective, clients can access the wisdom of their parts without being run by them. This is true with all parts in the OC subsystem as well, especially, in the beginning, with OC protectors, keeping in mind that these parts are often less cooperative and more in need of trust-building experiences. With OCD, we need to be a little more careful with what comes next in IFS, befriending protectors. Befriending allows parts to relax in the knowledge that they've been heard and understood. We communicate that we are not trying to get rid of them and actually appreciate their intentions even if we would prefer to take a different tack. But with the *obsessional* managers, we need to be mindful that understanding doesn't lead to engaging in their stories either to justify or argue with them. Accepting that they are motivated by good intentions is very different than listening to or engaging with their drama, which can frighten other parts. These two processes, unblending and befriending, correspond to many of the mechanisms at work in evidence-based treatments for OCD.

Principles at Work in Unblending

Various evidence-based OCD therapies use concepts similar to blending and unblending, employing techniques that foster perspective-taking, such as defusion, decentering, emotion regulation, reappraisal, and release from inferential confusion. These have been shown effective in reducing OCD symptoms. Using IFS for OCD facilitates these beneficial effects.

ERP: Using the Experiments to Facilitate Unblending

As detailed in Chapters 2 and 6, "blending is the act in which a part takes over a person's seat of consciousness, or Self" (Schwartz & Sweezy, 2020, p. 281). Blending occurs on a continuum, from parts obscuring a little bit of Self to entirely taking over for Self, as often happens in OCD. The IFS concept of unblending involves helping parts become differentiated enough from Self and one another to allow the Self to be in the leadership role, offering greater clarity and perspective. In practice, unblending works much like methods used in family therapy sessions, where Richard Schwartz originated the technique. Therapists, when they notice a strong agenda, can ask the part—or suggest that the client ask the part—to pause or step aside, much as in family therapy the therapist can ask a family member to step out of a conversation or stand by in a waiting room (Schwartz & Sweezy, 2020).

But what if the part does not want to unblend? Often, with OCD, obsessional managers who are wary and hypervigilant, itching to put the subsystem in high alert, are extremely reluctant to risk potentially catastrophic results they believe will happen if they stand down. They do not, at first, relinquish their central position willingly. The client may feel highly identified with or aligned with the obsessional viewpoint, especially if OCD is severe. To help the OC managers recognize and give Self a try, IFS therapists will do some contracting with them, negotiating some space or speaking with parts and Self directly to demonstrate the disparity. As Martha Sweezy (2023, p. 23) explains,

> . . . all parts need to be in relationship to the client's Self. Protectors don't have to do anything about this beyond being willing to stop doing what they do. When they stop doing and stand by, the Self shows up, which drains their drive to keep doing. But if this is to happen, they need direct experience with the Self. We may need to start with little experiments before protectors stop working.

Here, IFS and exposure principles are aligned. There often needs to be an intentional and significant experience for parts to learn something new, an exposure to the feared experience. So, Self-led ERP often begins with, "Would that part be willing to let you try?"

In the beginning of therapy or when a client has minimal access to Self, we find that starting with even the smallest sliver of curiosity, a willingness to try something relatively easy, can open the door to more Self-energy and facilitate further unblending. Alongside this invitation to try an experiment, which is usually offered to the obsessional manager, it's wise to also make an agreement with the firefighters who function mostly at the insistence of OC managers. We ask the firefighters if they would be willing to do an experiment too and pause before jumping in with compulsions, so that we can see if there might be another way. In other words, we do a trust-building exercise that ERP would call response prevention.

OCD experts usually encourage jumping quickly into exposures. And in this way, that is what IFS for OCD is suggesting as well. Although the "deeper" exposures occur in Stage Two, everything we do is experiential and involves encounters. This begins with the trust-building experiments in Stage One and continues through the ongoing engagement with triggers in Stage Three.

Defusion from Self as Content: Unblending to Differentiate Parts

Defusion and Self as Context are central concepts of ACT and have demonstrated value in OCD treatment. ACT addresses patterns of perceiving and interacting with the world that have become problematic and limiting; it is used regularly in the treatment of OCD (Hayes et al., 2003). ACT encourages psychological flexibility and detaching from rule-governed behavior by using defusion.

Fusion—a concept similar to blending—is defined as (p. 32):

> [an] excessive attachment to the literal content of thought that makes healthy psychological flexibility difficult or impossible . . . it draws the focus of living away from the present moment into the past and the future.

Defusion is a cognitive, intellectual process that helps people observe thoughts and feelings rather than becoming absorbed in them. This promotes experiencing self as the *context* for thoughts and feelings rather than their *content*. While defusion and unblending create similar differentiation, with unblending the client becomes aware of the part generating the thoughts and feelings. With that comes recognition that the part has developed with a good intention: to either protect a vulnerable part, so the person doesn't experience pain, or control other protective parts that might be more disruptive (parts that act out).

Decentering and Mindfulness: Unblending to Shift Perspectives

Unblending in IFS also maps onto *decentering*, one of the mechanisms at work in mindfulness processes (Comeau et al., 2024). When parts unblend, clients step out of living *as* their parts and shift to being in relationship *with* those parts, which changes the level of emotional disturbance they wield. Being able to say, "That's just a part of me," means the client knows and feels that the part is *not* "me, who I am." Stepping out of an immediate, blended experience and disidentifying from the internal state reduces the tendency to be reactive to the content of a troublesome thought.

This shift resembles the extensively studied mindfulness mechanism of *decentering* (Comeau et al., 2024), which involves (1) metacognitive awareness of subjective experience, (2) disidentification from that experience, and

(3) reduced reactivity to its content (Bernstein et al., 2019). Lebois et al. (2015) found that mindful attention showed greater activity in brain areas associated with perspective shifting and effortful attention, while immersion showed greater activity in self-processing and visceral state areas. This suggests mindful attention produces decentering by disengaging embodied self-sense from imagined situations, preventing affect development.

Self-related processing pertains to the complex "self" construct widely studied across disciplines. Several psychological models propose that mindfulness training shapes self-related processes, including self-regulation, self-efficacy, and self-concept. These concepts are cornerstones of IFS therapy and key to its effectiveness for OCD.

Emotion Regulation and Reappraisal: Unblending for Self-led Regulation

Emotion regulation is the ability to influence one's own emotional state by altering both the process of emotion generation and its expression, both of which are important factors in the escalation of anxiety and compulsive de-escalation seen in OCD. Many approaches to regulating emotions are effective. Some are healthy, and others are not as beneficial. Parts-led emotion-regulation efforts (compulsions) are experienced as effective in the short term but ultimately make OCD symptoms worse. These parts-led efforts include safety behaviors such as modifying or avoiding a situation, paying attention selectively, or using distraction. These methods tend to call on compulsive firefighters who are effective, but at a cost. Other forms of parts-led emotion regulation common in OCD include both rumination and thought suppression.

More adaptive regulation focuses on cognitive change such as *reappraisal*, a key concept in CBT, which involves the modification of the meaning that people make of their experience. In IFS, unblending is comparable to reappraisal and many of the 8 C's are involved in this process. Reappraisal is a healthy and stable form of cognitive change through which people achieve emotion regulation. When therapists help a client notice that a strong thought or feeling is coming from "a part," that move is a reappraisal of the experience, making it less all-encompassing and mitigating some of its impact. This shift allows the person to be present with and even curious about the internal experience rather than identified with it, thereby enabling a sense of agency, which opens an opportunity to work with the experience in a variety of ways. Distance enables perspective-taking, which emotion-regulation research recognizes as more adaptive than experiential avoidance strategies. Through unblending IFS offers a highly relatable, experiential way to achieve this clarity without it becoming a cognitive intervention that can run the risk of turning into a compulsion.

Principles at Work in Befriending

In traditional OCD treatment, clients are usually encouraged to fight back against their OCD. OCD is often framed as a monster or bully, and the client is encouraged to stand up to it, and not to let it win. This point of view works in the context of standard ERP therapy, but IFS takes a different approach. IFS aligns with the more paradoxical principle of leaning into rather than resisting. In all relationships, we can often take the power out of a struggle by first understanding the motivations of the other side. So, IFS for OCD involves befriending our OC protector parts in order to help them relax.

Because OCD sufferers have been told that OCD plays tricks on them, they have learned to be highly suspicious of their own thoughts and feelings. Identifying and befriending these "tricky" OC parts allows clients to cultivate an understanding of them while maintaining an inner knowledge of, and trust in, Self. The ability to detect a part is developed through a process of engagement: *not* by ignoring the part, *not* by just noting it and moving on, and *not* by letting it drop. Rather, befriending is a process of acknowledging the presence and good intentions of protective parts, while remaining simultaneously separate from, and curious about, them. As always with OC parts, we focus on the part and its motives, not the content of its concerns or the stories it tells.

When IFS therapists help clients with OCD befriend their parts, we help them develop Self-to-part internal relationships that foster a sense of security and the ability to trust themselves. With Self in the lead, clients are able to stay close and connected to a part without identifying with, or becoming overwhelmed by, its thoughts, feelings, or sensations. Self leads, not follows, the part. Befriending is a process of connecting with parts in an open-minded and understanding way. It does not mean that the therapist and client engage with the content of a part's concerns, reason with it, or prove it right or wrong. Rather, our goal is to learn the nature of the part, what it does for the client, and what drives it. The questions we ask are designed to explore the motive for the reasoning process that underpins the doubts, vulnerabilities, and fears that the part protects. When the part feels as though the client's Self can honestly say, "I understand why you think you need to do that, and I have similar goals, so let me help," the part sees that the therapist, the client, the Self, and the part are all on the same team. When this happens, the therapist is in a position to ask if the part would be willing to let all involved reach that common goal another way, by helping the exiled part directly.

Self-Compassion

The concept of self-compassion has recently been found to be a valuable adjunct to standard ERP because it defuses the self-critical attitudes that often get in the way of clients performing their assigned exposures and maintaining their motivation to continue treatment. In her *Self-Compassion Workbook for ERP*, Kimberley Quinlan recommends accessing compassion before and during traditional exposures, and she offers many methods to do so (Quinlan & Hershfield, 2021). But clients sometimes find it hard to purposefully be more compassionate toward themselves. IFS helps by offering another road to compassion through releasing constraints and softening the parts—often internal critics—that get in the way.

The Reasoning behind Obsessional Doubt

Like I-CBT, IFS for OCD facilitates the client's ability to hear and understand an obsessional narrative from a Self-led perspective rather than becoming absorbed in the story's potential to be true and the emotional impact of that possibility. Using different languages, both approaches encourage an evaluation of the reasoning from a present-centered and process-oriented perspective.

I-CBT posits the root of OCD in *inferential confusion*: a state of mind that occurs when the client's reasoning process is grounded in a distrust of external sensory data, internal sensory data, and common-sense ability to put internal and external reality together (O'Connor & Aardema, 2013). Similarly, IFS for OCD recognizes that when the client's obsessional managers have blended, clients see the world through the eyes of the part. Clients make moves based on the fear messaging of the part that is inferentially confused and therefore can't tell the difference between reality and feared possibilities. With befriending, IFS fosters Self-to-part relationships in which the therapist facilitates a shift from speaking *from the part* to speaking *for the part* acknowledging that "a part of me may feel like I have to wash, but I know otherwise." Clients are encouraged to understand the intention of the part in order to disarm it much like I-CBT teaches clients to understand the logic and reasoning behind inferential confusion. Learning to first differentiate, and then trust, the information that comes from the Self in the present world of consensus reality is done through understanding the process without getting entangled in the content.

Stage Two: Witnessing and Retrieval

In Stage One of IFS for OCD, therapists help OC protector parts pause, recognize Self, and trust enough to give the therapist and client permission to approach the exiles, effectively brokering a relational version of response prevention. In our discussion of Stage Three, we will return to these protectors to help them adjust and practice.

Stage Two is the Self-led ERP version of exposure and begins by shifting attention toward the encounter with the exiled part that holds the scary possibilities for the subsystem. Traditionally, exposure therapy involves engaging in an anxiety-provoking experience or contacting a stimulus in a *certain way* that involves not avoiding or eliminating it, but approaching it with curiosity, openness, awareness, and contact with the present moment. With that definition explained, IFS lead trainer, author, and therapist Martha Sweezy (personal communication, November 19, 2021) affirmed— "Everything we do in IFS is exposure."

The healing steps in IFS, used here in Stage Two of Self-led ERP, are designed to help the exiles feel seen and heard by Self, so that they no longer have to flood the system to be recognized. Not until they are fully witnessed can they let go of their burdens, including the feared possibilities that they hold as certain ("I am bad") or uncertain ("What if I'm bad?") options. When exiles unburden, the feelings and negative beliefs are able to dissipate freeing up the attention of Self to respond to life with more flexibility and the full range of a person's capacities. The IFS healing steps that are most closely related to exposure principles and therefore pivotal for transforming the OC subsystem as a whole, are witnessing and retrieval.

Witnessing and Retrieval

Whereas ERP intentionally provokes distress and emphasizes getting through it, the IFS model supports a highly relational encounter with a distressed part that begins with compassionate witnessing. Witnessing is the process of being with the part it as it shares its painful experiences, feelings, and beliefs. In Self-led ERP, witnessing may occur as part of a deliberate move toward an external trigger (exposure) or as an intentional approach toward internal triggers (imaginal exposure). For instance, once a protective part—shouting warnings such as *Be careful!*, *Don't get too close!*, or *You need to wash that!*—has felt the presence of Self enough that it becomes willing to pause its urgency, the therapist may suggest turning toward the feared experience, thus engaging the part that the OC protectors are afraid of or averse to.

Retrieval is an important step because exiled parts get suspended in time the moment they are banished from awareness. This part of a person's personality doesn't grow or develop as time goes by. Although the fears of exiles feel very real and very current when they blend, after unblending the client's Self is able to see them with some objectivity and recognize that their emotions are out of touch with current reality. But these parts are stuck in a state infused by doubt, fear, stress, and confusion and they need to be consciously addressed and intentionally invited to shift.

Principles at Work in Witnessing and Retrieval

As an intentional blend of the valuable healing aspects of IFS with the evidence-based methods for OCD treatment, Self-led ERP recognizes and relies on the commonalities underlying these seemingly different approaches.

Exposure: Witnessing the Exile from Self

Most of the conventional approaches to OCD are exposure-based and experiential: Clients are to reorient themselves toward their experiences, suspend avoidance and safety behaviors, and find the courage to just see what happens. When exposure therapy works, clients discover that the feared outcome didn't happen: They learn something new about themselves and the world. Now they can respond rather than react.

Witnessing in IFS involves the same principle, but is focused inside, on a part that holds the fears, distress, and uncertainty that protective parts are working to avoid. Like ERP, when witnessing with an exile, protective parts are asked not to interfere. So, the process involves encountering the exile (exposure) while protectors refrain from interfering (ritual prevention). But here, framed in the highly tangible and relational language of parts, Self asks parts who may want to jump in with compulsive attempts to alleviate the distress to step back and allow the exile to be fully seen, heard, and experienced.

Mindfulness and Self-Compassion–Based Exposure: Witnessing

Mindfulness has been well accepted in the field of OCD treatment because, as Jon Hershfield explains, mindfulness *is* exposure, because it similarly involves the choice to be in the presence of whatever arises internally or externally, including triggering thoughts or feelings, without judging or neutralizing them (Hershfield & Corboy, 2020). Mindfulness forms a critical link from OCD treatment to the methods of IFS because witnessing is mindfulness, infused with both compassion and reciprocity.

The Feared Self and the OCD Bubble: Retrieval and Unburdening

I-CBT pointed out that, although the content is not the issue in OCD, obsessions are not entirely random either. They tend to be organized around a theme of vulnerability they call the Feared Possible Self. This is an entirely imagined possible future identity that a person fears and dreads becoming. It represents their worst nightmares about who they might be, and often triggers intense anxiety and compulsive behaviors aimed at preventing this feared self from materializing (O'Connor & Aardema, 2013). From an IFS perspective, this is not a part. It is the negative self-referential belief or the burden that a vulnerable part has taken on. This is the reason that the part has been exiled: Other parts find it a horrifying possibility to be avoided at all costs. Stage Two of IFS for OCD is designed to bring attention to the difference between the part and the burdens, allowing the negative beliefs to be released.

Obsessional reasoning occurs and thrives in an imaginary world separated from the current reality. The OCD Bubble is an inferentially confused state of imaginal absorption in which all of the feared possibilities seem real (O'Connor & Aardema, 2013). Like this bubble, the exile's world differs from the client's real world. These parts feel stuck in a different time and place and retrieval helps them return to the client's current reality. Once the part's predicament has been witnessed and fears acknowledged, we ask if the part would like to leave the place and time in which it took on these burdens. Often the part has never considered this and is relieved to leave the past. The connection with the Self breaks the imaginal absorption in the obsessional content and offers another way for exiles to feel secure besides having protectors jump in with their safety solutions. Realizing Self's calm confidence is new for exiles who have previously relied only on protectors.

Stage Three: Reconnecting with Protectors

After facilitating this encounter between the client's Self and the exiles, we will help the OC protectors—and any other protectors who are involved—adjust to the inclusion of exiles in the subsystem. This requires a shift from being organized around the idea that exiles (and their feelings) are intolerable to an acceptance that they just needed their feelings to be felt. Often this requires some rehearsal of connecting to Self in the present moment in which we ask parts to try doing things differently. This third stage helps the client reengage in life activities that had been given up because of OCD.

I discovered the importance of this stage through my work with many clients who reported that their OC protectors didn't want to stop. Many clients said, "It is like they are on autopilot" or "The part says it is just what they do." In IFS, if this happens, we generally suspect that part is still motivated by an exile it is protecting, and that may be true for many in OC subsystems as well. As this approach evolves, I am discovering that, regardless of whether the motivation is coming from an exile or an unchanged, sticky brain circuit, these protectors continue to need attention and help in order to accept and adapt to a new, less extreme role in the subsystem.

Update, Engage, and Integrate

The updating of OC protectors after exile unburdening begins at the end of Stage Two, which includes some integration and appreciation. It becomes more explicit in Stage Three when OC protectors typically need extra attention to accept that they can lower their guard and can trust Self. Here we bring parts up to speed, creating new connections and associations to the present reality.

Stage Three takes the internally secured gains out into the world, showing protectors what Self-leadership looks like in action. Like the process of inviting lost qualities back to exiles, experiencing the intrinsic satisfaction of new freedom invites protectors to see new options. We invite them to try something new: engaging in previously inaccessible life activities. Research shows (Apergis-Schoute et al., 2017; Vaghi et al., 2017) that safety learning is particularly challenging for people with OCD. One single experience may create ongoing fear that drives OC protectors for years, but it often takes more than just the experience of the exile unburdening for the protective system to generalize that safety across situations. An exile might release a burden from a specific time, but since then, protectors have repeatedly frightened other parts, creating countless burdens in various situations. Generalization of safety requires practice and repeated opportunities for Self to show up, helping protectors build trust.

Integration happens when internal and external worlds receive balanced attention. Self-led ERP facilitates return to previously avoided activities, and OC protectors witness Self-leadership results, including increased security and confidence despite unproven safety. Over time and with practice, OC protectors' trust deepens, and they more readily accept new engagement possibilities when lowering their guard.

Principles at Work in Updating, Engaging, and Integrating

Stage Three begins after the exiled part or parts have been attended to in some way and to some extent. This does not mean that exiles have been fully retrieved, unburdened, and healed, just that there has been a successful encounter in which the client's Self has been able to welcome these parts and demonstrate to protectors that they will not overwhelm. The return to protectors in Stage Three is where this learning is solidified, reinforced, and begins to generalize to more real-life experiences. As this begins to happen, confidence is increased and willingness to continue becomes more robust and shared by more parts.

Using IFS in this way promotes the mechanisms of change that make ERP, ACT, and I-CBT so successful with OCD, and it adds the relational, and security-enhancing features of IFS.

Inhibitory Learning: Updating Protectors about the Encounter

The inhibitory learning approach to ERP emphasizes the role of *expectancy violation* in the ERP experience. OCD specialists recognize that a valuable aspect of the process is for the client to make the explicit connection that although many parts of the person expected something dreadful to occur, it did not. Even for those whose OCD is not focused on a disprovable event, it's helpful to emphasize that the feared feelings were not only tolerable, but that the parts who were holding them also have been lovingly accepted. The client now knows, experientially, that the beliefs that drove those feelings are not true. *Updating* occurs as part of integration at the end of the healing steps in IFS, and we elaborate this process in IFS for OCD during Stage Three. An update is when the client sends a message to all parts involved that there has been a shift. Usually, this means that Self is more available and there is no longer a need for the extreme work of protective parts. Taking the time to be sure each part with OC-related concerns has registered that Self can be with the previously scary feelings without the interference of protectors reinforces the trust.

Acceptance and Willingness: Integrating the New Relationships

IFS for OCD spends time in Stage Three helping protective parts adapt to new internal dynamics: Self leads, and the exile, no longer experienced as dangerous, has been welcomed back. As discussed in Chapter 5, ACT involves six processes designed to help clients develop psychological flexibility (Self-leadership). The capacity to be flexible facing uncertainty without rigid rules and behaviors is what Stage Three of IFS for OCD develops.

The ACT principle of committed action helps clients identify values to motivate and guide treatment. Rather than a cognitive exercise, IFS's final stage offers all parts the opportunity to rely on the organizing features of a Self who considers all internal perspectives. Choices to navigate formerly challenging experiences and engage in previously avoided activities can be trusted because they come from Self. Protective parts may still object: They may be unaware an exile was safely encountered or fully healed. Once updated, they still often need proof they can trust Self and relinquish extreme roles. They may need practice in various situations, but when Self chooses valued activities, these experiments feel meaningful. Because fear learning is durable and generalizes while safety learning decays easily and doesn't generalize, continuing to build Self-to-part relationships through meaningful activities is important to secure parts transformation and prevent relapse.

Reality Sensing and the Real Self: Rehearsing Self-Leadership

Stage Three of Self-led ERP helps clients build a strong, secure connection to authentic Self even when OC protectors are active. I-CBT highlights differences between true Self and obsessional narratives. Reality sensing points out disparities between the external sense-verifiable world and the imaginary possibility world in the OCD Bubble. When clients become more connected to their sense of Self rather than fearful parts' partial views, the whole system functions with greater freedom and clarity. In Self-led ERP, updating protective parts and appreciating their efforts while practicing engaging in Self-led courageous choices dismantles the OC story's impact without dismissing the part constructing it. Like I-CBT, the goal is helping clients return to trusting their senses and sense of Self in all areas—even those typically OCD-triggered.

The Big Picture

Using IFS for OCD in three stages I've called Self-led ERP creates an experiential therapy in which we maintain the features of empirically supported approaches that have been proven effective with OCD and infuse them with the compassionate and personalized, experiential methods of IFS. Of particular value is that we can intervene in a number of ways that have been proven effective with OCD, and we can do so in the depathologizing language of parts and in the spirit of befriending. First, at the very beginning of the OCD cycle, we can intervene at the level of the obsessional doubt sequence, leaning on the methods of I-CBT. Using IFS principles, we get to know the obsessional managers who experience inferential confusion and engage in obsessional reasoning, and we begin the process of unblending, in which parts become more differentiated from Self and one another. Next in the cycle are the parts who hold the distress, and the ones who fix it. IFS for OCD allows us to also intervene with the exiled part holding the distress and, in the service of response prevention, help compulsive firefighters refrain from ritualizing. In this way, we are also utilizing the exposure principles of ACT and ERP, and we are doing so with compassion and mindfulness.

Another benefit is that we can focus *internally* and perhaps heal some of the parts involved in precipitating factors that may have sparked OCD symptoms in someone already predisposed. And we can also focus *externally* helping a more Self-led client engage in valued life activities. In this way, we are also addressing the perpetuating factors that reinforce OCD. Self-led ERP was designed to recognize that the cornerstone of effective OCD treatment involves exciting the fear system and allowing it to regulate itself without compulsive, neutralizing actions. But this does not need to be done harshly in the spirit of deliberately provoking distress and training managers to tolerate it. When an exile is activated, we do have to help compulsive protectors pause long enough for Self to step into the leadership role, but IFS for OCD establishes a secure internal system of parts with harmonious relationships and a compassionate Self who is empowered to take the lead.

With the flexibility to apply various proven mechanisms as appropriate for our client, with the IFS goal of increasing Self-leadership at the forefront of our minds, we help clients develop the autonomy and self-efficacy that reinforces treatment gains going forward.

References

Apergis-Schoute, A. M., Gillan, C. M., Fineberg, N. A., Fernandez-Egea, E., Sahakian, B. J., & Robbins, T. W. (2017). Neural basis of impaired safety signaling in Obsessive Compulsive Disorder. *Proceedings of the National Academy of Sciences, 114*(12), 3216–3221. https://doi.org/10.1073/pnas.1609194114

Bernstein, A., Hadash, Y., & Fresco, D. M. (2019). Metacognitive processes model of decentering: Emerging methods and insights. *Current Opinion in Psychology, 28*, 245–251. https://doi.org/10.1016/j.copsyc.2019.01.019

Comeau, A., Smith, L. J., Smith, L., Soumerai Rea, H., Ward, M. C., Creedon, T. B., Sweezy, M., Rosenberg, L. G., & Schuman-Olivier, Z. (2024). Online group-based internal family systems treatment for posttraumatic stress disorder: Feasibility and acceptability of the program for alleviating and resolving trauma and stress. *Psychological Trauma: Theory, Research, Practice, and Policy.* https://doi.org/10.1037/tra0001688

Hayes, S. C., Strosahl, K., & Wilson, K. G. (2003). *Acceptance and commitment therapy: An experiential approach to behavior change* (Paperback ed.). Guilford Press.

Hershfield, J., & Corboy, T. (2020). The mindfulness workbook for OCD: A guide to overcoming obsessions and compulsions using mindfulness and cognitive behavioral therapy (2nd ed.). New Harbinger Publications.

Lebois, L. A. M., Papies, E. K., Gopinath, K., Cabanban, R., Quigley, K. S., Krishnamurthy, V., Barrett, L. F., & Barsalou, L. W. (2015). A shift in perspective: Decentering through mindful attention to imagined stressful events. *Neuropsychologia, 75*, 505–524. https://doi.org/10.1016/j.neuropsychologia.2015.05.030

O'Connor, K., & Aardema, F. (2013). *Clinician's handbook for obsessive-compulsive disorder: Inference-based therapy.* Wiley-Blackwell.

Quinlan, K., & Hershfield, J. (2021). *The self-compassion workbook for OCD: Lean into your fear, manage difficult emotions, & focus on recovery.* New Harbinger Publications.

Schwartz, R. C., & Sweezy, M. (2020). *Internal family systems therapy* (2nd ed.). The Guilford Press.

Sweezy, M. (2023). *Internal family systems therapy for shame and guilt.* The Guilford Press.

Vaghi, M. M., Vértes, P. E., Kitzbichler, M. G., Apergis-Schoute, A. M., Van Der Flier, F. E., Fineberg, N. A., Sule, A., Zaman, R., Voon, V., Kundu, P., Bullmore, E. T., & Robbins, T. W. (2017). Specific frontostriatal circuits for impaired cognitive flexibility and goal-directed planning in obsessive-compulsive disorder: Evidence from resting-state functional connectivity. *Biological Psychiatry, 81*(8), 708–717. https://doi.org/10.1016/j.biopsych.2016.08.009

Winston, S. M., & Seif, M. N. (2017). *Overcoming unwanted intrusive thoughts: A CBT-based guide to getting over frightening, obsessive, or disturbing thoughts.* New Harbinger Publications.

Winston, S. M., & Seif, M. N. (2019). *Needing to know for sure: A CBT-based guide to overcoming compulsive checking and reassurance seeking.* New Harbinger Publications.

Part IV

The Practice of IFS for OCD

Self-led ERP

Chapter 9

IFS-Informed Assessment of OCD

As we have seen, Internal Family Systems (IFS) theory explains how and why protective parts in general are motivated by the well-intentioned drive to keep the painful burdens of exiles out of awareness. As these burdens become more intense, protective parts must take more extreme measures and behaviors to achieve their goal. That's why relieving the exiles' burdens is enough to help many systems come back into balance.

With obsessive-compulsive disorder (OCD), however, neurobiological differences, combined with life experience and other factors, intensify the relentless nature of the parts that trigger, exacerbate, and maintain symptoms. For this reason, and because it's possible for therapy to aggravate rather than help clients with OCD, it's always important, when obsessions or compulsions are noticed, to begin treatment with a thorough OCD assessment. While most IFS therapists integrate an ongoing assessment within their usual process, an initial assessment (Pampaloni et al., 2022) is necessary when therapists suspect OCD, because IFS treatment will require a different path, one I call "Self-led ERP," which can reframe exposure and response prevention as *encounter and relate to parts*.

The practice of IFS for OCD—Self-led ERP—integrates empirically supported OCD assessment and treatment with the IFS mindset. This union sets the stage for successful results by establishing a compassionate understanding of the symptoms and helping the client's parts feel confident that they are understood. When using Self-led ERP, we adapt the traditional OCD assessment methods described in Chapter 4 to the non-pathologizing language and unique assessment tools of IFS described in Chapter 2.

Some clients may come to therapy with clear symptoms of OCD, but many clients whose symptoms fall into some of the less-common OCD subtypes don't realize the nature of their distress. Instead, they may feel that there is something uniquely and drastically wrong with them. Especially when they experience themes of harm, or intrusive thoughts with themes of sex or violence (which are often accompanied by mental compulsions rather than overt rituals), clients often are terrified not only by

DOI: 10.4324/9781003449812-14

their thoughts but by the very fact of having them—as well as fears about what the thoughts may mean. An accurate diagnosis accompanied by psychoeducation is the first step to providing compassionate relief for clients with OCD, many of whom may have gone for years or even decades feeling scared of their own minds and without effective understanding or help.

In combination, the OCD symptom assessment and the IFS assessment work together to gather relevant information about obsessions and compulsions. Integrating these two approaches allows us to see the functional relationships between obsessions and compulsions more clearly as the work of obsessional managers and compulsive firefighters. In addition, the combination has therapeutic benefits: As we take our clients systematically through traditional OCD checklists and scales, they may feel immediate relief, understanding—perhaps for the first time—that the urges and behaviors that are making them feel uniquely "crazy" are, in contrast, well-understood symptoms of a known disorder. And as we work through these inventories using the lens of IFS, we use the information about symptoms to get to know our clients' parts, their jobs, and their fears. Where the typical OCD inventory, for example, has statements indicating whether a thought "troubles me" or more complete statements such as "I have aggressive thoughts or impulses" (Myers et al., 2008), we apply an IFS perspective to reflect back that "a *part* of you has aggressive thoughts." This translation of standard OCD assessment into "parts language" usually feels revelatory to people with OCD, as the vast majority will tell you that those thoughts do not represent what they truly want, feel, or believe.

However we choose to begin assessment in Self-led ERP, the manner in which we approach our questions sets the tone for the therapy to come, and so we model compassionately attuned curiosity as we explore the whole system of the person in front of us, the dynamics of the person's OC subsystem, and the relationship of the subsystem to the whole—as well as the complex relationships among our clients' internal systems and the external systems (family, work, etc.) that they inhabit. In the process, the quality of our presence provides clients with a sense of security that supports the therapy to come.

This chapter illustrates the process of assessment in Self-led ERP, following the structure of the OCD assessment process established in Chapter 4, infusing each step with the approach and language of IFS. After elaborating on the two IFS assessment questions as they apply to OC subsystems, this chapter applies them to the gathering of relevant history, functional impairment, symptom inventories, and the collection of information about triggers and insight. In this chapter, I primarily illustrate the process using one case example, that of Aracelli. Going forward, the remaining chapters of Part IV alternate among a variety of partial case examples as they clarify the various concepts discussed.

Applying IFS Assessment to OCD

IFS engages the whole experience of the client in order to understand the situation that brings the client to therapy. Initially that includes assessing for safety and capacity to benefit from therapy as well as support or constraints in the external environment. It's a global and continuous process that takes in a person's whole internal system, including strengths and capacities, viewing the presenting symptoms as the understandable efforts of parts operating within a plurality of internal experiences (Schwartz & Sweezy, 2020). Understood in this way, symptoms themselves hold valuable information.

Because OCD seems to operate as its own subsystem of parts and their relationships, understanding the client's whole internal system in which the OC subsystem is embedded brings to light both a person's internal supports and capacities in relation to OCD as well as other parts that may interact more critically with the OC subsystem. In other words, the larger system may have strengths and strategies that already exist and can be recruited to help in conversation with the OC subsystem. Conversely, there may be challenges presented by other important issues that need attention prior to or alongside OCD. Understanding the larger system also sets the stage for helping parts who have taken on extreme OC roles to be absorbed back into more harmonious roles and relationships.

In the usual process of IFS treatment, assessment occurs throughout. Beginning with noticing and understanding parts that are present in the moment and gauging access to Self by paying attention to how much blending versus differentiation the client experiences, it becomes increasingly nuanced as it unfolds throughout the phases of treatment. Still, in essence, it's a simple two-pronged process:

> IFS assessment generally revolves around two questions. First, we want to know if the symptomatic part or parts (e.g., depression or anxiety) are protectors or exiles. Second, we want to know how much access a person has to the Self.
> (Schwartz & Sweezy, 2020, p. 101)

Does This Part Have a Job?

As we listen to our clients with OCD, it's likely that we will hear from many parts that will eventually need our attention, some OC related, some not. Still, it's likely that an OC part will need our attention fairly soon, becoming one of our first target parts. When any part becomes a focus of attention, we work to understand its role and get to know its function by asking our first assessment question: "Does this part have a job?" Parts *with* jobs (protectors) shield a person from distress and parts *without* jobs (exiles) hold the distress. If the target part has a job, it is a protector—a manager or a firefighter. Since obsessions and compulsions are defined by their functions—increasing or decreasing distress—this is a particularly relevant question in the Self-led ERP assessment of OCD. OC parts with jobs are the ones creating the symptoms; OC parts without jobs are the focus of these activities. Sometimes when we ask the target part whether it has a job, the answer is no: It just says things like, "I feel ashamed" or "I'm scared." In that case, the part in question is an exile: It's just there with its feelings, to a greater or lesser extent.

Once we discover how a target part participates in an OC subsystem, we'll know more about how to approach it. By relating to the OC protectors (the ones with jobs), we set the stage for the "RP" part of ERP by helping them pause and recognize Self. Parts without jobs need attention, so we will move toward them compassionately to encounter those parts in an IFS version of exposure, the "E" of ERP, orchestrated through the IFS healing steps.

As a rule, like regular IFS, IFS for OCD begins therapy by getting to know protectors. But if the part that requires immediate attention is an exile, we may initially engage with that part in order to build trust and ask it not to flood the system while we get the protectors on board. Occasionally, we might engage more extensively with the exile presenting its strong feelings upfront. Whether we can do this depends on the willingness of the protectors to step back, which, in turn, depends on how much access the client has to Self. This leads us to the next question.

How Do You Feel toward the Part?

The more qualities of Self a client can access (curiosity or clarity, for instance), the more open to therapy the client can be. This determines how fast or slow we will proceed. With OCD this can be challenging because OC managers doubt that there is any other way to be sure to avoid disaster besides their system of recruiting or compelling firefighters to act. Because the therapeutic process is supported by the compassion, curiosity, willingness, and courage of Self, determining how much access there is to Self and when and how that awareness becomes obscured by parts is one of the most potent benefits of bringing IFS to OCD treatment. Is the client open and curious when a strong part is present? Or blended with the target part or a part that is reactive to it? We gauge how much Self is available by noticing body language, pacing, tone of voice, and eye contact. For example, a client with OCD may recognize a part whose job it is to keep the person's whole system on alert by pointing out potential dangers. We would then ask the second assessment question, "How do you feel toward the part?" The client might calmly say, "It's interesting to see it like this. I wonder what made it so frantic." Because we hear one of the 8 C's—curiosity—an indication that Self is available, we know we can guide the client in a relational dialogue with the part. If, instead, the client avoids eye contact, freezes up, and says, "I just know I have to do things in a certain way, or I'll be anxious all day," we know that the client identifies with the part and its feelings. They may also say that they hate the part or feel intimidated by it, in which case we would point out that there is another part in the driver's seat—one with strong feelings who will either try to eliminate the target part or acquiesce to it. Either way, Self is not in the lead; the client is blended with a part. This is the work of Stage One of Self-led ERP, helping the part to unblend so the client has access to Self.

The IFS-Informed OCD Assessment

Whether we start traditionally with an OCD checklist or we start in an IFS manner with the parts that show up, using IFS for OCD involves using our knowledge of OC parts from the formal assessment tools to inform our curiosity as we seek to understand both the dynamics of the person's OC subsystem and the relationship of the subsystem to the whole. Specifically, we interview parts about their background and relevant history, including concerns about functional constraints; symptoms of OCD, including safety-seeking behaviors; severity of symptoms; and prompts and triggers. Throughout, we pay attention to the person's level of insight into fear of consequences of exposure to triggers without engaging in compulsion.

Background and Relevant History

Understanding the situation from both an IFS perspective and an OCD perspective means that we are interested in both internal and external constraints. *External constraints* is the IFS term for information about limiting factors in the client's outer life including current stressors, physical safety, substance use or addictions, the role and nature of family members, socioeconomic facts, and relevant cultural information. *Internal constraints* may include the residual impact of past traumas or burdens that are rooted in life experience, any dangerous firefighter activity such as suicidal parts, and parts that are invested in blocking change. Understanding both the internal and external systems that are currently affected or may have been affected by OCD or previous treatment for OCD is how we begin to develop a treatment approach that holds both the relational and the behavioral approaches.

Aracelli, for instance, had both successful and unsuccessful experiences with traditional exposure therapy prior to our work together. Because of her trauma history, it was clear that gaining trust would be key to our own treatment: Her parts needed to learn that they could trust me as well as ultimately trust her Self. Much of the progress she had made in previous treatment attempts unraveled, even though, as she reported, she had done everything asked of her. One part of her believed that these relapses meant that something was so wrong with her that she would never get better. By exploring what other parts had to say, we discovered that some protectors had not agreed to the treatment plan and were undoing the interventions as they were happening—unbeknownst to her former therapist. Getting to know which parts were not on board allowed us to develop more trust in the current process. Letting these parts know that they could speak up if they had concerns so that we could move at the proper pace gave us a clear sense of how parts were responding in the moment and made them less likely to undermine treatment. This allowed Aracelli to engage more fully.

Symptoms of OCD: Obsessions and Compulsions

Far from being pathologizing, assessment and diagnosis of OCD help clients recognize what their parts are doing and why. Most clients feel relieved, appreciative, and hopeful once they recognize that they are not uniquely stuck and alone. With IFS for OCD, we recognize obsessions as the work of OC managers sounding alarms and compulsions as the work of OC firefighters remediating the situation to quiet the alarm. Exiles are the parts that hold potentially dangerous feelings or beliefs. Although they are the ones that presumably all the fuss is about, they are not the cause of OCD or even the perpetuating factor. Seen this way, traditional OCD assessment and the IFS model can be used together very productively. Clients' parts who may have been in hiding often feel seen and acknowledged in the process of going through an OCD checklist together, and parts engaged in obsessions and compulsions may relax a little by simply being recognized.

As we have seen, IFS clinicians have learned over time that certain parts show up on a regular basis in IFS therapy, parts such as critical managers and indulgent firefighters. Listening for parts commonly found in OCD will be part of the assessment process. Likewise, with OCD, we commonly see a specialized set of protectors who engage in the thoughts and behaviors listed on any OCD checklist. We will notice parts that function as scanners, assessors, alarmists, checkers, and remediators to name a few. Some of these parts amplify distress and others neutralize it. As clients with OCD begin to differentiate and flesh out those parts with their particular characteristics, they become more attuned to the differences between their own OC parts and their sense of Self.

A key nonpathologizing feature of IFS is its convention of supporting clients' natural tendency to spontaneously attribute demographic qualities such as gender and age to the parts, and to give them descriptive names such the runner or the hider, and even personify them as, for instance, "my Mean Coach" or "the Scolding Woman." These names add layers of description that create a sense of the part as more than just its extreme role. Including the client's personification of their parts in our assessment demonstrates our respectful and relational stance toward their good intentions, and at the same time, facilitates a convenient conversational shorthand for referring to the client's complex OC thoughts, feelings, and behaviors. For instance, Justin had an extreme hypervigilant scanner that he described impersonally as "the Wary part." Eventually Justin began to call it "the Watchful Guy," because it—now "he"—sounded like an older brother, maybe even a father, who just wanted Justin to be careful. As his relationship with this protective part became even more personal, Justin found he had more agency to ask the part to pause or soften his tone, and the part began to see Justin as the older figure, and that Justin was there to take care of *him*. A role reversal had occurred in which Justin began to see the part as younger. Eventually, the young Watchful Guy softened and revealed his fears so that Justin was able to access the exiled part he was protecting and help that part release its burdens. Naming and describing the part allowed Justin to notice it before it got too intense and pulled him in to an OCD spiral.

Exiles show up in assessment as the feelings that the client is trying to manage or eliminate. They too, may be given personal names, such as "Terrified Gracie," in which the client is using her own name and referring to the feeling she can't stand. Sometimes, names indicate a more amorphous part, such as The Gross Blob, referring to a part burdened by a feeling of disgust or being dirty. For clients with OCD who may have spent a lifetime avoiding the feelings carried by these parts, recognizing them as belonging to a sympathetic part of themselves can allow for a greater capacity to include uncomfortable feelings without needing to compulsively neutralize them first. This can make the assessment process also a hope-building experience in which the prospect of sitting with difficult emotions becomes more meaningful or tolerable.

These obsessional and compulsive protectors have their counterparts on most standard OCD checklists, so the common IFS practice of what we call developing a good "parts map" with a client can be an adaptation or supplement to doing an inventory. (As explained in Chapter 2, a parts map is a method for visually representing a client's parts and their relationships.) However, clinicians who are not as familiar with OCD should review several standard OCD inventories so that when these characters show up they ring a bell. In addition, sharing OCD inventories with our clients can be a helpful way to begin to provide psychoeducation, which sometimes has a surprisingly unburdening impact almost immediately with clients who had not previously understood their OCD. Using IFS, we would frame the items on an inventory as the activities of parts, and the endorsed items on these lists can help identify parts that will need unblending. We can immediately begin to map them to set up the contract for therapy. By creating a clear picture of the parts involved, we facilitate the client's parts in seeing Self and beginning to unblend.

For instance, Aracelli came to therapy already having completed a variety of OCD inventories. Still, when we discussed them in the context of parts talk, she appreciated seeing a visual representation of how parts with these concerns were interacting.

Many of Aracelli's obsessions and compulsions revolved around questions of potentially being responsible for harm coming to her family. An OC manager shouted constant warnings and *what ifs*. If she didn't listen to these cautionary thoughts, another part jumped in to throw out multiple, horrifying images of her children, dead. These visual obsessions were so disturbing that they were usually the ones that rallied the compulsive firefighters to act. At first, we weren't sure if the same part was using both verbal warnings and images, but as she looked inside with curiosity, she found that the two tactics felt like they were coming from different parts. This became useful information later in treatment. She called one of them the "Scolding Woman" and the other "Emo Movie Guy" at one point. Her dawning recognition of these parts as centers of *motivation* rather than as a function of *content* allowed her to begin to befriend the parts without engaging or getting entangled in their content.

Severity of Symptoms

Assessing functional impairment is often accomplished by listening to parts with reactions to the OC subsystem. Many parts of a person may feel frustrated by the apparent needs of the OC subsystem and the lengths to which those parts feel compelled to go. Parts who are upset about OCD often start therapy by ranting about all of the reasons they want to "get rid" of the OC parts. It's important to be diligent about listening to these complaining parts, even as we keep track of, and maybe note out loud, how harsh or critical they sound. While upset parts will relax more easily once they have been heard, their initial frustration provides crucial information about how extreme the OC protectors have become, which informs our choices about treatment and possible referrals for the client. Hearing these parts out may be the best source of information about safety behaviors such as avoidances that may be quietly inhibiting progress toward freedom from OCD.

To get a sense of the internal limitations that prevented Aracelli from experiencing the kind of life she wanted to live, I asked her to tell me about a typical day. On most days, getting her children fed and ready for school was her first challenge, as she struggled to pack lunches for the children so that they wouldn't be late. Even after the children left for school, her own self-care was severely affected. Her day was consumed by making sure that she did everything until it was just right. She checked her purse—over and over—to be sure she had her keys and phone. She made lists; she wrote and re-wrote emails. She needed to make a plan for the day before eating or showering, which took so much time that sometimes she didn't shower at all. She often didn't eat until after putting the kids to bed at night. Her sleep was degraded because she needed to check on the children multiple times each night. These limitations would inform our approach in Stage Three when we help her engage in valued activities

Prompts and Triggers (And the Parts Who Find Them)

With OCD, anything can be a trigger, prompting an OC cycle, so it's helpful to identify particular items, people, situations, and even thoughts that are triggering for certain parts. For instance, a part who proactively manages potential contaminants for someone with contamination OCD might repeatedly steer attention toward certain items such as doorknobs, table tops, or trash cans, or toward ideas such as laziness or anything associated with negativity. From an IFS perspective, OC parts—usually obsessional managers—scan for, hyperfocus on and grab ahold of triggers and then elaborate them by telling stories about their potential ramifications, making meaning of their presence or otherwise sounding alarms. Clients often report experiencing obsessions as a two-step phenomenon. First comes an *uh-oh*, an awareness. Then, almost immediately, an obsessional part grabs the awareness and keeps stirring it up until a firefighter jumps in with a compulsive thought process such as rumination in order to soothe the system. A list of prompts and triggers can function as a road map for getting to know the parts that interact with them. The result of a transformed relationship with these parts is agency.

For Aracelli, as with many clients with OCD, numerous situations and events could make her feel panicky and new triggers could pop up at any time, but there were consistent ones that we could start with. For instance, food preparation and cleaning products were always challenging whereas being out with the kids could trigger random fears of losing her way, forgetting her belongings, or passing out and not being able to take care of her children or animals. When she didn't avoid these activities, she attempted to neutralize her fear by a great deal of anxious checking and repeating compulsions.

Level of Insight

Typically, when insight is considered poor, the outcomes of OCD treatment are negatively affected. In these cases, IFS is particularly valuable. The principles of blending with parts and unblending explain a great deal of this apparent inability to differentiate Self from OCD. By facilitating internal differentiation of parts from Self and building Self-to-part relationships once that differentiation is established, IFS for OCD helps clients develop a more clear sense of the differences between the voice of OCD and their own thoughts and feelings.

Unblending is a fundamental process in IFS throughout therapy, and it is an important aspect of assessment. How blended parts are and how many parts are blending at the same time as well as a client's awareness of parts all contribute to determining access to Self and ability to have insight. When exiles carrying distress flood the system or when protective parts are highly blended and burdened, the 8 C's qualities of Self are hard to access. Clients demonstrate very little clarity, and so insight is said to be low. While blending and unblending happen naturally all the time with everyone, the ebb and flow of parts is punctuated by the presence of Self and the accompanying C qualities. In an IFS-informed assessment of OCD, we determine insight as a function of blending and the intractability of the parts that have blended. This understanding is woven into the ways we inquire about OC symptoms and is highlighted by the second assessment question: How do you feel toward the part?

Standard OCD assessment often begins by asking clients directly about their obsessions and compulsions: What are their concerns and the rituals performed to relieve those concerns. This approach often elicits a response that reflects the clients' confusion between what Self knows to be true and parts fear to be true. They may say, "I have to check again even though I know I don't really have to," which highlights that both the Self and the part are involved and reflects some insight. Because the IFS method of query recognizes that there's a difference between what our clients know and what their parts think and feel, IFS therapists may handle these questions a little differently. We ask clients what their OC *parts* are afraid might happen if they refrain from doing their jobs, that is, sounding alarms or performing rituals, understanding that the initial answer may not come from the client's Self, but from a protective part.

Aracelli was immediately able to recognize that she, her Self, did not buy into the idea that she had to go to such extremes to ensure the safety of family members. This did not make the horrible thoughts and images less distressing but it allowed her to progress through treatment without as much shame and frustration. This increased access to Self allowed her to find compassion for herself and her parts in tough moments, which gave her the internal support to resist compulsions.

Benefits of IFS Assessment with OCD

With multiplicity as the model of mind, using the techniques of IFS therapy with OCD enables us to help clients to recognize both their obsessional doubts and their compulsive rituals as the motivated behavior of parts. Clients become increasingly able to help these parts unblend so that Self can step up and take the lead. Greater agency comes from recognizing obsessional doubt both as *not me* and as *a part of me*. As clients become more Self-led, obsessions become less like uncontrollable intrusions and more like noise from rambunctious members of the internal family, with the client's Self as the firm and benevolent guardian. Compulsions become less over-reactive and destructive and more like our loyal first responders who are standing by on semi-retired status, there to serve if really needed but not in extreme ways.

Transcript: Inquiring about Obsessive and Compulsive Parts

Therapist: What are your primary concerns?
Aracelli: Well, I have to check things over and over and it drives me nuts because it takes me hours to do things. But I am just terrified of missing something if I don't.

[There are three parts speaking here: (1) a firefighter who "has to" check, (2) a part that is bothered by the OC subsystem, and (3) an obsessional manager who is worried about missing things.]

Therapist: So you have a part that makes you afraid you will miss something and a part that pushes you to check and repeat things. Does that sound right?

[Therapist notes an obsessional part and a compulsive part.]

Aracelli: Yeah, and so I'm always terrified something will happen to my family if I am not careful enough. And then I check so much that I don't take time to eat or shower . . . It's all so embarrassing.
Therapist: So, there's a part of you that feels like it means something bad about you?
Aracelli: Yes, but I want to make sure you know all the details because if I don't tell you I won't get better.

[There is a lot going on, so the therapist slows it down hoping to promote some differentiation and perspective.]

Therapist: Let's pause and recognize all that is going on. I am hearing four of five different parts, I think. There is a part that warns you about the possibility that you haven't been careful enough *(obsessional manager)*, one who is terrified about how bad you'd feel if you missed something *(exile carrying burden/core fear)*, and another part that gets mad and embarrassed *(system-wide critic)* at the OCD parts that make you check and repeat things *(compulsive firefighters)* and wants it to stop. Then you mentioned another part that doesn't think I can help unless you tell me everything right now *(perfectionistic manager)*.

Aracelli's presentation was typical of clients who come to therapy for OCD. People seek an OCD specialist because they can't stop washing or checking or ruminating about a concern—managers and firefighters run amok. In the OC subsystem, this protector alliance creates a formidable Self-like structure that becomes more and more extreme: the protective solution for being flooded by exiles' negative beliefs, feelings, and core fears. This cycle can be clarified by a good assessment using either an OCD checklist with notes about the parts who are engaging in the obsessions and compulsions or a parts map informed by an OCD checklist. Clinicians can adapt their primary methodology to create a more personally relatable roadmap for treatment.

This hijacking of Self by the efficiency of the OC protectors is the key feature in the progressive nature of OCD and an important reason it's imperative that OCD be identified and addressed. This cycle is difficult to stop without help. The following three chapters demonstrate the importance of supporting protective parts as they begin to take the risks entailed in trusting Self to make the call. These risks catalyze healing by empowering the system with the internal sense of security that comes from trusting Self. But first protectors have to be willing to try.

References

Myers, S. G., Fisher, P. L., & Wells, A. (2008). Belief domains of the Obsessive Beliefs Questionnaire-44 (OBQ-44) and their specific relationship with obsessive–compulsive symptoms. *Journal of Anxiety Disorders*, 22(3), 475–484. https://doi.org/10.1016/j.janxdis.2007.03.012

Pampaloni, I., Marriott, S., Pessina, E., Fisher, C., Govender, A., Mohamed, H., Chandler, A., Tyagi, H., Morris, L., & Pallanti, S. (2022). The global assessment of OCD. *Comprehensive Psychiatry*, *118*, 152342. https://doi.org/10.1016/j.comppsych.2022.152342

Schwartz, R. C., & Sweezy, M. (2020). *Internal family systems therapy* (2nd ed.). The Guilford Press.

Chapter 10

Stage One
Relating to Protectors and Accessing Self

Describing his first experience at a meditation retreat, psychologist Mark Epstein remarked,

> I always assumed that whoever it was that was doing the thinking inside my head was the real me. When I shifted my awareness in meditation, so that I was observing my thoughts instead of being run by them, it felt like a revelation to me.
>
> (Epstein, 2014, p. 89)

This is the crux of unblending in Internal Family Systems (IFS) therapy and the beginning of relating differently to protective parts in the obsessive-compulsive (OC) subsystem.

My reframing of exposure and response prevention (ERP) therapy as Self-led *encounter and relate to parts* creates a clinical mindset in which, depending on our training and the needs of the client, we are infusing conventional ERP therapy with the IFS approach or infusing IFS with ERP principles.[1] Self-led ERP utilizes a blend of IFS tools and exposure techniques to facilitate access to Self and trust in Self-leadership with the goal of helping OC protectors willingly relax into more moderate roles. Understanding the mechanisms of obsessive-compulsive disorder (OCD), therapists can use IFS techniques in an OCD-informed way to get to know parts without running the risk of reinforcing the OC cycle by engaging in reassurance or getting entangled in their stories.

This chapter explains and demonstrates how to use Self-led ERP to introduce parts and *parts work* to clients and begin the process of helping their challenging protectors unblend. It begins with the IFS approach to getting started in a therapy session, then offers specific tools particularly useful in the unblending process with OCD. With these foundations in place, this chapter lays out the steps of Stage One of Self-led ERP, illustrated with transcripts of the case material we've been following.

Before We Start

While overall Self-leadership is the ultimate goal of IFS for OCD, helping obsessional and compulsive parts pause their intense dedication to their extreme roles so they can feel the presence of Self is the focus of Stage One of Self-led ERP. Getting to know these protectors and normalizing the intrusive thoughts is how we begin to facilitate differentiation from them. The more differentiation that parts have from Self and from each other, the more choices become clear and the more it becomes possible to approach exiles and the difficult feelings they bring with them.

At the beginning of IFS therapy, protective parts determine how fast or slow we will go. From the perspective of traditional training in OCD treatment, getting into exposure as soon as possible is ideal. Whether that actually accelerates recovery is a question posed by many people who seek IFS therapy for their OCD. For those who have experienced some backlash after ERP, or who are afraid to attempt it, time spent with protectors building trust is certainly worth while. By checking in with our own parts and their agendas, we can be clear that we are finding the balance that best serves our client. Keeping exposure principles in mind as well as the IFS framework of befriending protectors, we do both. We encourage experiments from the very beginning as a way of getting to know the protective system and as a valuable avenue to building internal relationships between Self and parts. In other words, with IFS we do exposures relationally; first to increase awareness of obsessional and compulsive protectors and next to help these parts feel the presence of Self so they can relax or at least agree not to interfere. The intention is to develop "response prevention" capacities at the beginning by "relating to OC protectors." By strengthening their ability to recognize protectors when they show up, clients become more able to tell the difference between being parts-led and being Self-led. When clients can relate to OC protectors differently, from a sense of Self, the whole system can sense a shift. There is a recognition, even if only momentary at first, that Self can handle things without the compulsory interference of parts. This realization helps both to free the parts from their extreme roles and to restore trust in Self. The stronger these relationships are, the better.

The IFS mindset that "all parts are welcome" may not resonate with clients initially. The concept of befriending parts may sound odd or even outrageous and dangerous to other parts—and maybe even to some readers. We may be hearing from parts that are resentful of the control that OCD has over the whole system, or that are afraid of it, intimidated by it, or even traumatized or terrorized by it. It is understandably difficult for a client to get curious about the potentially good intentions of a part that has become brutal about demanding compulsions. It is equally correct to have concerns about engaging with the content of obsessional parts and their stories. But once we acknowledge these concerns and suggest a wider, more inclusive perspective, this curiosity allows more access to Self by helping to disengage from the struggle. The fewer internal voices clamoring for attention, the more clarity is available when we turn toward the OC protectors, and eventually, the exiles they protect.

So, after an IFS-informed OCD assessment (described in Chapter 9), we get to know the parts that show up first. These are often the parts that have strong reactions to OCD: self-criticism and judgment, anger and frustration, or intolerance of the extreme distress it can cause. I often hear clients say, "I know it's ridiculous but I have to. . ." or "it's really embarrassing but. . ." and other derogatory statements about their behaviors. This internal battle not only further entrenches the parts involved, but it adds to the internal noise and anguish. IFS for OCD begins by helping these parts release or at least soften that struggle. This is the first important difference between Self-led ERP and standard ERP, which often capitalizes on the energy of the parts who want to get rid of OCD. Exposures are often done *from* a part determined to fight OCD, and this can be helpful. But many clients find that without their angry parts and their internal critics chiming in, they can be more present and clearer as they get to know what the parts with the obsessions and compulsions are doing and how the cycle maintains itself.

Stage One: Relating to Protectors and Accessing Self

Step 1: Helping system-wide protectors unblend.
Step 2: Helping OC protectors unblend.
  Find, Focus on, and Flesh out.
  Check Feelings toward OC protectors to assess for Self-leadership.
  BeFriend: Ally with protectors; inquire and discover their roles and intentions.
  Identify Fears: What does the part fear would happen without it doing its job?
Step 3: Getting *enough* permission to go to the exiles.

Step 1: Helping System-Wide Protectors Unblend

Because Stage One is about accessing Self and building Self-leadership, our primary move is to facilitate unblending at all levels—from the system-wide protectors who are reacting to the OC subsystem to the specific

OC protectors within the subsystem. Although individuals with OCD are often angry or frustrated with their OC parts, they are also very accustomed to being blended with them. So, it sometimes takes time to help clients recognize their parts and settle on a place to start. They may first need to unblend from non-OC parts to get to know the fierce OC protectors with some compassion.

With OCD, parts that are critical of OC behaviors or frustrated and angered by these parts are common. So are skeptical parts that worry that the horrid obsessions may not be OCD talking but could be due to the person's actual moral failings, careless spreading of germs, or other feared possibilities. Typically, we want to start with the protector who is most likely to shut down the therapy process. With OCD, frequently frustration (another version of self-criticism) and intimidation or fear of OCD will get in the way, and so a critic or scared part is often the one who needs our attention first.

Aracelli's Frustrated Protector

In the exchange below, we see Aracelli becoming able to address a part of her that is frustrated with OCD. The part is getting in the way of us encountering her OC protectors in an open-minded and curious way, and we ask it to unblend.

Aracelli: [*Her frustrated manager speaking.*] This keeps happening and I'm really trying not having these thoughts. I know it's just my mind. It's me getting into my head and just thinking about all these alarming things. Like I think, "He could die." And then I really *feel* like something's going to happen. And I'm really wanting to make sure it's not going to happen. It's a never-ending cycle. It's frustrating and I hate that I can't be more easy-going.

Therapist: Would the frustrated part be willing to step back so we could get to know the part that's terrified that your son is going to die?

Aracelli: Well, but having those thoughts all the time just makes me a little bit . . . I just get angry. It's so unnecessary. I hate my brain. I just want to get better

Therapist: [*Acknowledging the frustrated protector who needs to be addressed.*] Ah, I get it. I can see why that part of you is mad. That's probably the part that brought you here, is that right?

Aracelli: Totally.

Therapist: [*Encouraging befriending.*] This may seem odd at first but see if you could let the frustrated part know that you understand. You see its point, and that's why we're here.

Stage One: Relating to Protectors and Accessing Self

Aracelli: OK . . . Something shifted.
Therapist: *[Asking the part to unblend.]* Great. Try asking if it could give us a little space, so we could get to know the part that is telling stories about the safety of your kids. If it will give us some space, we could help that part.
Aracelli: I don't know . . . I'll try . . . Yeah, it can do that.
Therapist: Is the part who is sounding the alarm still there?
Aracelli: Always.
Therapist: How do you feel toward it now?
Aracelli: I wonder what it's doing. *[A response of curiosity, indicating the presence of Self.]*

With the ability to observe a feeling, such as frustration, and see it as coming from a part—disidentifying from it—comes increased access to Self. With access to Self comes all of the 8 C's qualities of Self-energy, although usually not all at once. Here, and often, we see curiosity first, but eventually, this process leads to compassion toward the OC parts and the ability to acknowledge their good intentions as well as how hard they've been working. When Aracelli was feeling frustrated toward her OC parts, we stopped and acknowledged the frustration until that part felt heard and was able to release its grip on her attention. Once it did, we were able to turn our attention to the OC parts that created the symptoms that brought her to therapy: obsessional doubting and compulsive neutralizing of that doubt and uncertainty. With the more open-minded clarity that comes from unblending, Aracelli was now in a position to turn toward the parts in the OC subsystem. Shaming, critical parts are often some of the first to show up, and they are persistent. Continuing to address these internal critics as needed makes room for the compassion that will support the process.

OC Adaptations of IFS Tools for Unblending

When hypervigilant OC managers insist on putting the system on high alert and are certain that to relax would create a high likelihood of threat, they understandably have a hard time letting go. Because OC protectors are notoriously reluctant to unblend, Self-led ERP utilizes the usual IFS moves with a few twists and adaptations. In the very beginning, we may first be helping parts that hide, hate, or are afraid to go near OC parts, but the processes are the same. We routinely use the conference table, mapping, and other externalizing techniques described in Chapter 2, but contracting and experimenting are worth addressing here in an OC-specific way.

Contracting with OC Protectors

IFS therapy sessions generally begin with a contract for where to focus, which evolves in the course of a session. After we check in with clients to see what parts are present at the moment, we ask them to see which of their noted parts needs our attention first. Once the target part is clear, we ask the client to check in and see if any other parts might object or have concerns about us addressing it. This query can get dicey with OCD but it's still an important step. OC subsystems often have a lot of parts with concerns and one of them might want to make sure that all of them are heard "just right" or completely. We use our clinical judgment to discern when to turn to a part demanding absolute completion and firmly ask it not to interfere or ask it what it would need to give this process a try and allow us to turn to an OC part.

Experimenting to Access Self

If contracting doesn't create the amount of space you need to proceed, you can ask parts if they would be willing to pause as the client turns toward something frightening or uncomfortable with curiosity—a small, incremental experiment. The intention here is to create an opportunity for a part to meet Self. Using the language of "experiment" lowers the sense of risk for protectors and can increase the likelihood of their willingness to engage. When the therapist and client get buy-in from OC parts to participate in a small experiment, the client's whole system has an opportunity to see and feel more Self-energy, which facilitates further unblending and encourages other parts to agree to experiment, too. It's usually easiest to begin with the compulsive firefighters who are engaging in obvious physical rituals, but any protector, a skeptic, for instance, can choose to step back and give permission to try a small experiment.

Step 2: Helping OC Protectors Unblend

Obsessional managers and compulsive firefighters are the guardians of the OC subsystem, so these protectors are generally our primary focus in Step 2, which is essentially an OCD-specific application of the 6 F's. We spend some time becoming familiar with these parts without arguing with them, engaging in their stories, or increasing their investment in their efforts by opposing or pushing them away. Reducing the over-responsibility of OC parts dedicated to keeping the OC subsystem "safe" takes patience.

This time spent getting to know obsessional managers and compulsive firefighters has two purposes. First, it helps the client more easily recognize OC protectors when they show up and facilitates the ease of future unblending. Second, it is a relational way of getting protector buy-in for "response prevention" so that backlash is less likely. As with ordinary people in our lives—who listen better if we have listened to them first—acknowledgment is disarming for parts. They respond to being recognized, loosen their grip, and become more willing to unblend. This process allows a connected but differentiated perspective that soothes a client's anxiety because it acknowledges and accepts the client's obsessional managers and compulsive firefighters as they arise, and it does so with the compassionate and confident presence of Self. The key is to acknowledge that the OC protectors are motivated by something and have good intentions, and also to suggest that they have another option, which is to allow Self to take the lead. Tailoring our approach to what we hear from the parts, we come from a place of curiosity and compassion.

In Stage One of Self-led ERP, we follow the IFS 6 F's with OC parts to help them unblend:

- First, we *find* the part. This search involves helping clients tune in to the one part that needs attention first, the initial target part. We guide them to notice trailheads—the thoughts, feelings, sensations, urges, or images that provide clues to their inner states and lead to parts, and their drives, needs, and motivations.
- Next, we *focus on* the part, noticing how it shows up in or around the body so we can connect with it rather than just think about it.
- *Fleshing out* is the process of helping clients become a little more acquainted with their experience of the part and learn to feel a differentiation between the target part and Self.
- After we have settled on a target part and clients notice its differentiation from Self, we guide them to check how they *feel toward* the part. This helps us gauge their access to Self.
- When clients feel one of the 8 C's toward the target part, we are in a position to *befriend* it. Here, we inquire more into the job the part does for the OC subsystem. With OC parts we need to be careful not to get involved with the obsessional content: We are getting to know the part, not its stories.
- Finally, we inquire to *find its fears*. Again, these are not the obsessional fears themselves, but what the part fears might happen if it let go of its job.

Find, Focus on, and Flesh out with OC Protectors

We begin with the first three steps of the 6 F's. (Because they flow naturally from one to the next, I have combined them for Self-led ERP.) After we ask clients what parts they are noticing in the here and now, we follow the trailheads. If just one part is clamoring for attention, we go with it. If there are many (which is often the case), we ask another simple question: "Which part needs your attention first?" If there's a clear answer, that's our target part, and we help that part to differentiate and recognize Self. If the answer is murky or bounces around among multiple parts, we continue to listen and reflect parts back to the client as we hear what the parts are up to, perhaps using a conference table technique or mapping to help many parts unblend and create space for Self. Sometimes compulsive parts show up and need attention first, but often an obsessional manager wants to begin. We follow what seems most pressing to the client, knowing that these parts are all related to one another, and we will meet them in due time.

Justin's Roadblock Protector

In earlier sessions, Justin had wanted to address his contamination fears in the bathroom but had gotten too overwhelmed by terror to proceed with ERP. So, we began to use IFS techniques to build a connection with the parts that were getting in the way. Finding the parts of himself that were blocking him from facing his fears wasn't difficult once we made it clear that it was not our intention to change them. As Justin internally imagined a typical day, he noticed a number of trailheads, bodily sensations that led him to the awareness of parts. After he found several different parts at work—an alarm-sounding scout, an avoidant controller, and a critic—Justin chose the one he called "the Scout" as the initial target part to focus on and flesh out. Closing his eyes, he focused on how he felt this part's presence. He reported that the part stood very close and directly in front of him, also looking forward but blocking his view of his day. It was as if the part was a parent guarding a child under its protection. The part had its arms out and wouldn't budge. As Justin paid more attention to its presence, he became aware that it wasn't shutting him down for no good reason. It was on the lookout for danger. Justin became more attuned to how the world looked through the eyes of this part with whom he had been identifying, and by taking a step back to see the part more clearly, he began to notice all the small choices he made throughout the day from the viewpoint of this part. By getting to know the felt sense of this part on a sensory level, Justin was able to notice this part more easily when it would show up and to separate its views from those of his own.

Aracelli's Bossy Mom Protector

Once Aracelli's frustrated part stepped back, we moved into Step 2 by finding, focusing on, and fleshing out the initial OC part that had presented itself.

Therapist: So can you focus on the one who needs your attention now?

Stage One: Relating to Protectors and Accessing Self

Aracelli: A part of me is afraid that Matthew's going to die from eating something that isn't well prepared at school. I know he wants to eat cafeteria lunches like his friends, and I want him to have that experience. But a part of me is terrified. I get these awful images of him choking and keep thinking, "It would be your fault. You could have sent him with safe food." The thoughts and images taunt me. It's awful. *[Aracelli was a natural at speaking for parts rather than from them.]*

Therapist: Do you want to pay attention to the part that sends those thoughts and images?

Aracelli: Yes, it's happening right now.

Therapist: Can you check inside? Close your eyes if it helps, and just notice where and how that part shows up, in or around your body? *[Find.]*

Aracelli: It's mostly in my head, shouting at me, and showing me horrible images.

Therapist: What else do you notice about it? Does it have a certain tone? Can you see it? How close is it? How big or small? *[Focus on and Flesh out: Here I'm helping Aracelli experience her obsessional part as different from her so she can recognize it more easily. Notice that I am not focusing on its story or arguments, and I mirror her use of the pronoun "it."]*

Aracelli: She's like a small, bossy mom in my head. My actual mom was never paying attention back then so it's odd, but that's what I see. *[Following Aracelli's shift in pronouns, we'll use the word "she" and the name "Bossy Mom" when we discuss this part later on.]*

Through this exchange, Aracelli began to sense the part as separate from herself. Noticing details such as the quality of the voice or a feeling of pressure or—if the client is good at visualizing—how the part appears is extremely valuable because it helps the client develop an impression of the obsessions as "not me, but a part of me." The client becomes more adept at catching the thoughts or feelings of parts as soon as they show up rather than immediately identifying with them. Now instead of thinking, "*I have to*" or "*I can't*" the client can think "*This part* is telling me what to do."

Scott's Quality Controller

Scott wanted to start with a part he called his "Quality Controller," a part that never let him rest and unrealistically overestimated what he should expect of himself. Operating under these OC mandates caused Scott to feel overcome by shame if he even considered taking a "short cut" to anything.

When Scott and I began to speak, he was blended with his Quality Controller part, saying "I need to know that I am doing the best I possibly can." When prompted to find and focus on his target part, Scott was able to locate it physically on one side of his head. After checking with Scott that it was OK to explore a little more, I suggested he try to describe the part, to flesh it out. "How does it show up?" I asked. "Is it mainly a thought, or does it also come with sensations or a visual?" In locating and describing that pressured voice, Scott became aware of the physical effects of listening to the part: Hearing its voice made him lean forward, feeling tension all the way down to his stomach. We now had access to Scott's Self who was able to notice the part when it showed up and was also surprised to notice it so clearly. Once Scott tuned in, he was able to hear what the part was saying to him.

Scott: I hear this voice that says, "Wait! Are you sure that's accurate? Did you represent yourself fully and are you sure those are your words? Maybe you're plagiarizing. You'll get caught and expelled and your life would be ruined!" *[Scott is still leaning a little forward and bringing his hands to his head.]*

Therapist: Are you able to notice your posture and how this part is showing up right now?

Scott: Wow, yeah . . . this part is intense!

Therapist: See if you can take a step back and really notice what it looks like, how you feel it and what it sounds like, how big it is and any other details. *[Fleshing out.]*

Scott: It's kind of like a giant. It dominates and gets in the way of any relaxation or fun.

Scott described a common OC protector experience; that his Quality Controller was unrelenting and immovable, and wrecked his ability to rest. He was unable to have fun with his friends, or even finish his work on time, which ironically sabotaged the good intentions of the part. Understandably, he had other parts who hated it. We continued to need to help those parts step aside as we continued with this part so that he could see it from a place of more differentiation and with curiosity and compassion.

Feel Toward

Before clients get too deep into conversations with an OC protector, we want to first make sure they have enough access to Self and are not communicating *from* a part. Compassion and curiosity are key components in this work because a thought we are battling often becomes more intense and intractable. But simply *wanting* to be compassionate doesn't always

Stage One: Relating to Protectors and Accessing Self

work. So, IFS therapy facilitates access to Self—signaled by any of the hallmark 8 C's—by identifying what is getting in the way. By asking how the client feels toward the target part, we notice other parts that have strong feelings or agendas and then we can ask them to step back: A lot of feelings may be standing in the way of Self, so we address them all one by one, and we keep checking until all of the parts that are reacting to OCD in that moment have relaxed or stepped away. We check back every time we sense that these reactive parts may have returned—one of the main ways in which IFS therapy is recursive rather than manualized.

When the client has more space internally, natural compassion emerges, and the client can focus on parts that identify as core parts of the OC pattern. In this way, the parts that most need to meet Self can do so, and a true internal encounter can proceed, one in which the OC parts feel heard. This understanding, this compassionate connection that creates true willingness to encounter core fears, arises out of some recognition of and trust in Self.

Scott's Interfering Parts

Asking Scott "How do you feel toward that part?" opened the door for him to access the Self-energy necessary for getting to know his Quality Controller and its unyielding demands on him. But first, it also invited participation from other parts that might be as yet unrecognized. Finding background participants is important for therapy because they're frequently the ones who get in the way of connecting compassionately with the target parts.

Therapist: How are you feeling toward this giant part as you notice its huge and solid presence?

Scott: I'm intimidated and kind of angry. I really hate that it has so much power to block my way.

Therapist: I can imagine. You have parts that are understandably daunted by this big guy. *[Parts detecting and facilitating unblending.]* Can you acknowledge the angry one, and then ask it to let you handle the giant? Let it know that if we can help it soften it will be better for all your parts.

Scott: OK, I don't feel as angry but I still feel intimidated because the Quality Controller can really pull me into a spiral fast.

Therapist: That's good to know. Let that intimidated part know that we hear that, and I am confident that we can get to know this part without letting it take over. *[Addressing the protector fear of overwhelm. Note that this is not a reassurance accommodation because we are not complying with a compulsive firefighter demand. We are helping a part who is blocking therapy to feel more secure and allow us to proceed.]*

Scott: OK ... that's a little better.
Therapist: How do you feel toward the Quality Controller now?
Scott: I see him as a kind of a lumbering giant who just wants to do his job. He doesn't seem as mean or harsh as he did. *[Without other parts in the way, Self is able to see the softened version of the part.]*

Scott wouldn't be able to truly see the Quality Controller's good intentions when coping with the parts that were afraid and angry jumping in. When we asked these scared and angry parts to step back, we emphasized that doing so would not allow the Quality Controller to take over (their main concern) but that it would have the opposite effect by creating more space inside for Self. When we heard Scott's curiosity we were also checking for other indicators of Self—his tone of voice, body language, etc.—and to see if any other parts were still there. Since the intimidated one was still present, we helped it have more trust in Scott's Self so it could relax. When scared parts trust Self, the scary parts seem less intimidating.

BeFriend

Befriending OCD instead of battling it is a curious concept—especially since so much of OCD treatment has long been framed as a heroic fight against a relentless OCD monster or bully. But befriending is an essential part of Self-led ERP: Especially with a part that's causing problems, we want to get to know and understand the part and its motivation to help it let go, not to react or respond to its argument.

In the spirit of IFS, we do not *prevent* OC protectors from doing their jobs; instead, we befriend them and persuade them to take a break. Viewing parts as internal centers of motivation, it makes sense that when we acknowledge them and appreciate their intentions, they are less combative and more willing to hold back on their OC activity for the time being. We ask them to pause for long enough to see that Self is able to contact and experience the exiled part and the feelings and fears that come with it. The result is that the client and the client's whole system have a new, more positive experience, learning that OC protectors are not the only safe option, that, in fact, Self offers a more secure and flexible approach. When these protectors have a relationship with Self and are seen as a valuable part of the internal ecosystem, their transformation is more reliable over the long term. (We address the particular nature of OC protectors after unburdening in Chapter 12, where we discuss Stage Three of treatment.)

Befriending OC protectors in this way, getting to know them with an open mind, is not the same as conceding, making the best of it, or naïvely saying "it's all good." Rather, befriending OC protectors involves committing to a *transformational* level of acceptance and respect for all parts, even ones that are hostile or dangerous or otherwise extreme. It doesn't mean we engage in a discussion or try to understand or get to the root of what the part is saying, just that we see that it is doing the only thing it knows how to do at the moment, and we appreciate that it has a well-intentioned, even if counter productive, reason for its actions. With compassion, we are better positioned to offer it an alternative route to finding relief. When clients become able to befriend their OC parts, they become wiser and more capacious. They develop a steadiness that resounds throughout their system, and all their parts—OC and otherwise—respond.

There are some caveats about befriending with OC protectors, and so we need to be able to create kind but firm boundaries so that they don't take over. If the part is an obsessional manager, it may be connected to a low-threshold and "sticky" danger signal in the brain that the part may have erroneously associated with a set of circumstances. These obsessional managers are often described as switchboard operators who can very quickly activate the body and other parts with elaborate narratives to explain their actions and association. If the part is a compulsive firefighter, it might similarly decide to repeatedly demonstrate its ability to respond and its effectiveness.

Experienced IFS practitioners who are less familiar with OCD must be careful not to follow obsessional managers into discourse about the dangers they protect against. Questions about *why* a part does its job can lead directly to a validation of its doubts, thus reinforcing them. We don't want to focus on what the part *thinks*; we want to focus on its role and how it functions: What it does and what comes afterwards. Conversely, experienced practitioners of exposure therapy who are less experienced with IFS should note that although the therapist and client are connecting with an OC protector, the focus is on the *relationship* between the part and the client's Self, not on the content of concerns. This focus fosters the same supportive connection that is suggested to parents of children with OCD (Lebowitz, 2019), that is, acceptance in the form of a combination of compassion and confidence that the child both has big feelings and can survive them. Befriending their own OC parts in this parental spirit allows clients to compassionately understand the parts' function or motivation for sounding alarms without weighing in on the content. We will be alerted if we are interacting with a protector in a problematic way because the client's system will either calm down immediately—because a compulsion has occurred—or it will escalate quickly because we have validated its fears.

The compassionate but confident stance of befriending is natural when there is enough access to Self, which is why we ask how the client feels toward the part first. With feeling compassion and curiosity toward the part, clients are less likely to get into agenda-driven questioning that is designed to assess the validity of the obsession or ensure safety or reduce anxiety. Instead, we find the willingness to know and understand the parts and help them find some relief. This more genuine connection offers relief from the urge to battle with the part, which only fuels its investment in its position. This way, when the OC part senses that Self understands, it can relax its grip. Not surprisingly, we find that parts are more willing to step back when we are not trying to get rid of them or change them.

The IFS method of befriending an OC protector involves understanding what motivates the part to do what it does. Chapter 2 introduced the concept of *insight*. When a client's Self is able to hold a conversation with one of its parts, we can support the client's quest for insight by suggesting that *the client ask the part* questions and listen inside for a response. Questions can include:

- What's your job? What is it that you do for me? What are you hoping to achieve?
- How long have you been doing that job? When did you start doing your job?
- Are you working too hard?
- Do you like your job? Is there something else you rather be doing?
- Are other parts helping you? Getting in your way?

Asking questions such as these helps build a sense of connection, trust, and understanding between Self and part. Ideally, at the end of the befriending process, the client will be able sincerely to tell the part, "I get it now. I understand and I don't blame you for doing that. Let me see if I can find another way." They understand the reasoning behind the concerns. With Justin, *insight* was effective to establish a connection.

Justin's Scout

Justin wanted to speak with the part he had called the Scout.

Therapist: Are you aware of the Scout right now?
Justin: Yes. He's kind of always there taking stock of everything, looking for problems!
Therapist: Let him know you're here to help and notice how he responds.
Justin: Hmmm... He shook his head, like "no way." He's unimpressed.
Therapist: Ask him who he thinks you are. Maybe also how old he thinks you are.
Justin: Just someone young who needs his help.
Therapist: Maybe offer him an update. Show him who you are now, what you do, what life is like when it's working.

Justin: He registered that but has his doubts.
Therapist: OK. Ask him what he's doing for you. Just listen.
Justin: He says he has to take in every detail around me and keep track of everything so he can be sure I don't spread dangerous germs.
Therapist: How long has he been doing that for you?
Justin: Most of my life

By understanding the part's motivation, Justin could now appreciate the part for what sounds like a good big-picture goal of not harming others. Then from a place of alignment Justin can offer to handle that job a different way, with Self in the lead, deciding how to achieve it. Since Justin could now access more Self-energy, when he started to notice that he was feeling afraid of contamination, he could remind the part that he was in charge, bringing the part's attention to the present-day version of himself with an update. Helping the Scout recognize Self and remember that they are on the same team, Justin could calmly remind the Scout that he would make the decisions about what he touched on his own.

Find Fears

At this point, we are in a position to discover the fears that are the focus of the OC protectors. It's a core principle of IFS (including IFS for OCD) that protectors (even extreme OC protectors) believe that what they're doing is essential to preserve the person's wellbeing—whether that be love and acceptance, safety, or peace of mind. So, when we ask a part what it thinks might happen if it stops, or scales back on doing its job, it will respond with a fear. This fear describes what is at stake, the core fear of OCD, and points us to the part of the client that the protectors are dedicated to eliminating or exiling. (Unburdening those exiles is the subject of Stage Two of Self-led ERP, which we discuss in Chapter 11.) Once we know more about the fear or burden of the exile that organizes the OC cycle we know what the exposure/encounter will be: We'll encounter the part who has been exiled for its role in allowing this feared experience to crop up.

With OC protectors, it's good to be aware that obsessional managers who are sounding alarms or sending intrusive thoughts will usually provide a laundry list of terrible things that could happen, or horrible feelings that might arise, on a timeline that seems to stretch out to forever. Parts that are extremely hypervigilant may say that if they don't continuously scan for danger, the person may do something that will result in irrevocable harm. But listening to a protector delivering a tirade is *not* befriending. We want to discover what the part thinks it is protecting so that we can facilitate a release of the urgency through the presence of the Self. But with OCD, we need to be mindful of parts engaging in OC activity around this demand to be understood "once more time," or "just right"—in other words, on their terms. Engaging in such a conversation can easily slip into engaging in compulsions with the client.

Aracelli's Vulnerable Exiles

In some situations, multiple obsessional parts protect the OC subsystem from a single exile in somewhat different ways; in others, a single obsessional part protects more than one exile. For example, Aracelli has an exile who feels vulnerable as well as another one holding burdens of guilt and shame. The following exchange reveals the specific concerns of her obsessional Bossy Mom, a protector who has many concerns and subtle ways of getting her needs met, and who tries to keep both exiles out of awareness.

Therapist: Do you want to ask her what she's afraid would happen if she dialed down the intensity of all of those horrible thoughts and images?
Aracelli: She says that I would lose my focus and something devastating would happen. *[Vulnerability.]* And then I would feel awful—like it was all my fault—and I just don't think I could live with being someone who would allow that to happen. *[Guilt and shame.]* I know that's not going to happen, though. The kids will be fine. I can't protect them from everything. *[Another part jumps in, this time a compulsion to begin self-reassurance.]*
Therapist: Could you acknowledge the part that wants to reassure you and see if it would be willing to wait on the sidelines for a bit? *[Since we are speaking to the bossy manager, my first choice was to see if this compulsive firefighter would step back allowing us to continue negotiating with the obsessional manager for permission to help the exile. Had it put up more resistance it may have become the new target part and I would have returned to the beginning of Stage One, retracing steps 1 through 3.]*

As we begin to explore the fears of obsessional managers, we often find that other OC parts jump in to keep us from going there just like the system-wide parts that we mentioned in the beginning. This attempted intervention by one of Aracelli's compulsive firefighters provides an example of how important it is for the therapist to have a well-developed OCD-focused parts detector and the willingness to set a limit. Self-like and subtle compulsive firefighters can interfere without being obvious, stalling the process under the guise of being helpful. Had we engaged the firefighter with compassion and joined Aracelli in its reassurance, the obsessional manager would feel vindicated and Aracelli's anxiety would have gone down, but the alliance

Stage One: Relating to Protectors and Accessing Self   165

between these two parts would have been strengthened and Aracelli's Self would have continued to be excluded from the process.

When therapy feels stuck, it's often because the client's parts continue to engage in compulsions, sometimes surreptitiously, and sometimes even by maneuvering the therapist into participating in those compulsions with them. Knowing how learning happens and how patterns of reactivity are reinforced in the brain, we must recognize that each time a firefighter engages in a compulsive activity, the relief it provides to the OC subsystem—however small—reinforces the damaging conviction that this activity is necessary and effective, causing Self to remain unseen and unavailable to these parts. Here, again, we can be firm in a compassionate way. When I suggested to Aracelli that she didn't have to engage with the part attempting to reassure her, she was stunned:

Aracelli: You mean I should let myself think about what if the worst *did* happen?

Therapist: What comes up when you consider that?

Aracelli: If I don't convince myself that my kids will be OK, I'll have a panic attack. I'll start shaking and feeling dizzy. *[This is her bossy manager threatening again.]*

Therapist: *[I propose inviting her exile into the space.]* Maybe the one who thinks that would be willing to try something new. Would it like see how you'd handle it if the part that carries that panicky feeling was here with us now? *[We might not know which exile this is until we get to know it in the next stage of therapy.]*

Aracelli: Hmm. She's not sure about that but says she's willing to try if I think it's a good idea.

Therapist: What do you say to that? *[I avoid reassurance by not promoting certainty.]*

Aracelli: I want to try and see. *[Aracelli accepts some uncertainty and is willing to face the exile with openness and curiosity, i.e., Self.]*

As we get to know the obsessional concerns of a client's OC managers, easily recognizable firefighter compulsions such as reassurance-seeking, confessing, and remediating are not far behind. Often mental compulsions are putting out fires behind the scenes even during our sessions. In the assessment we most likely inquired about them specifically, but as treatment progresses, it's best to explore the ones that show up on their own and help the parts that are present begin to understand why they're quarreling with each other—if they are—or why they're aligned with each other if they have a common goal.

In Aracelli's case, this first stage of therapy helped her be more present, more Self-led, so that she was now able to recognize OC parts when they showed up and to let them know that she was available and present with them. Her parts became more willing to unblend and trust her, and Aracelli was ready to shift into the next stage of Self-led ERP: to connect with and heal the exiled part, eventually welcoming it back into the system as a whole.

Step 3. Getting *Enough Permission* to Go to the Exiles

This first stage of Self-led ERP aims to earn the willingness of OC protectors to meet Self and then to get their permission to shift our focus to the exile, but we acknowledge that this may taking some negotiating. An internal system that includes an OC subsystem may have multiple obsessional managers and compulsive firefighters ostensibly protecting against what is perceived as the intolerable threats of exiles. But in addition to the many typical protector fears about moving forward, OC protectors are likely also responding to neurobiology. This complexity means that you will almost certainly repeat the steps of Stage One with several parts before the OC protectors willingly pause their reactivity long enough for the client to truly encounter the exiles you've discovered. OC protectors rarely accept less than absolute certainty, which makes treatment more challenging. Even so, we can navigate this intensity skillfully with some patience and persistence, bringing our confidence to bear as well. With OC protectors, we ask that they be *willing enough* to give Self a try. Sometimes we need to be firm, knowing that the incremental efforts to demonstrate the efficacy of Self will pay off in the end.

That said, protectors, especially OC parts, may not show their full strength until we turn our attention away from them. When one softens, another may object. Since obsessional parts recruit compulsive firefighters, for instance, a firefighter who becomes willing to refrain from checking, for instance, may agitate an obsessional doubt part. That part may then up the ante and sound more alarms, with new thoughts, sensations, urges, or images. Similarly, obsessional managers may be able to pause only if a compulsive firefighter is willing to covertly remediate during the connection with the exile, undermining the connection with Self.

If one or both OC protectors jump back in after we begin to connect with an exile, we recontract and turn our attention where it is needed. Compassion and confidence as we relate with OC protectors facilitates more connected engagement with exiles, and therefore a more impactful exposure experience.

Scott's Persistent Firefighters

When compulsive firefighters show up in a session, are acknowledged, and become willing to unblend, they often lead us right to the exile who needs our help. When Scott, for instance, was able to help his ruminating part to pause, he was finally able to notice the shame it was distracting him from feeling. This realization is a choice point where therapist and client need to decide if it's best to shift immediately to working with the exile (an encounter with the shameful part) or to ask it to wait a while until we can give it our complete attention. If the protective system is willing to stay back and let us turn to the exile without compulsions interfering, we can proceed. If, however, the firefighter is insistent upon doing its compulsions, it's best to wait to avoid provoking a backlash. It's when we see a firefighter pause, soften, or step back that we have the clearest access to the exile it protects.

Sometimes we intuit the strong presence of firefighters who don't show up in session, but whose influence is keeping the client stuck. In such a case, we can return to the client's original assessment of compulsions and inquire about these parts. When something previously fearful doesn't seem like a big deal in the moment, we might ask if a part came in to help. This is often very illuminating and validating for the client.

When called for, for instance if the only way to get in touch with a part is to be in the triggering situation, we might use an *in vivo* encounter to help protectors see how Self handles the challenge. For example, if a client has Contamination OCD, we might ask protectors what they are afraid might happen if the client touched a railing or doorknob and refrained from washing or using hand sanitizer, and then ask if they'd be willing to test that hypothesis. Whether we ask clients to imagine a scenario or actually do something physical, they can usually access a part that says, "Awful! It would feel awful!" Here the therapist functions as a merchant of hope. We hold and present the possibility that if that action were possible and parts did not have to jump in to protect, they might get a break and the part who feels awful might get the attention it wants and needs.

Scott decided he would be willing to experiment by quickly posting something to social media during our session. After discussing options, he settled on a picture that he'd taken of a landmark on a recent vacation. His obsessional manager was doubting his certainty that it was his own photo: Maybe a friend had taken it, in which case it would be a lie to claim it was his. We helped the doubting part unblend so that Scott could feel a sense of Self. With more clarity, he was also aware of a second part that was critical of the worried one, saying it was a ridiculous worry, and another part telling him that he would be overwhelmingly stressed until he took down the post. Finally, a fourth part told him it would be OK because his therapist told him to do it, so if something went wrong, he wouldn't be to blame. Once Scott could identify those parts and we put them on a parts map, Scott decided that even if they didn't quiet down, he would like to try the exposure/encounter and see how it went. He posted the picture with an intentionally vague message. Then, we turned our attention to Stage Two: an encounter with the exiled feelings of dread and shame that arose immediately.

Welcoming

When we accept not only that all parts are welcome, but that they are also understandable, we are sending the message to those parts that we are trustworthy and on the same team. Generally, OC protective parts step back gradually and in shifts, so Self-led ERP is rarely as simple as getting a single OC firefighter to step back. But for that one firefighter, and for many of its peers, Stage One of treatment creates a foundation that fosters greater capacity for response prevention. By "relating to the protectors" who need to be on board for Self-led ERP to be successful, we create a natural, constraint-releasing stance that allows compassion to emerge on its own and, with that, the capacity to open to whatever the exiled part is holding.

With trust in place, we can move into Stage Two, the encounter with an exile. To be clear, this process is not traditional ERP, and so we are not simply doing an exposure to the feared trigger and then preventing the response or ritual. Because Self-led ERP takes a relational approach to a person's inner system, we first (in Stage One) acknowledge protectors and help them get ready to step back. Next (in Stage Two), we encounter exiles, and then (in Stage Three) we go back to reinforce relationships with the protectors. The new internal relationships mutually support inner differentiation and balance.

The healing encounter, in which Self is able to be with the exile and help to relieve its burdens, is how OC protectors learn more deeply that they can rely on Self-leadership. Usually, the obsessive manager is terrified of what might happen if the firefighter does not help, so asking the firefighter to pause and not do the ritual requires both OC protectors to have developed some willingness. Taking time in Stage One to develop that trust opens a path to Stage Two, in which OC protectors watch as Self courageously and compassionately encounters the dreaded feelings and experiences of the exile that protectors believed to be so dangerous and intolerable.

Notes

1 This approach also integrates principles from ACT and I-CBT. However, based on the viewpoint that much of what we do in IFS is exposure—in the broad sense of the word—and we are helping protective parts to pause_preventing rituals from occurring—the most accurate term continues to be Self-led ERP.

References

Epstein, M. (2014). *The trauma of everyday life*. Penguin Books.
Lebowitz, E. R. (2019). *Addressing parental accommodation when treating anxiety in children*. Oxford University Press.

Chapter 11

Stage Two
Encountering and Unburdening Exiles

"Absolution, after all, had a shelf life," wrote Shala Nicely (2018, p. 209) about her obsessive-compulsive disorder (OCD) rituals in *Is Fred in the Refrigerator?* With this poignant realization, Nicely encapsulated both the profound and fleeting nature of the relief provided by compulsions and, from the perspective of Internal Family Systems (IFS) therapy, by most protectors: Their efforts are effective in the short term but not transformational. That's especially true about compulsive protectors who work within an OC subsystem. Like many individuals with OCD, Nicely suffered from nonstop anxiety and doubt about a wide range of topics that made her feel vulnerable, irresponsible, guilty, and even as if her days were numbered. She found temporary relief from her anxiety by doing compulsions, but for those suffering exiles, security—when brokered by Self—is a more life-changing solution than the temporary safety chosen by protectors.

Stage Two of Self-led ERP, which augments exposure and response prevention therapy, is the process of encountering exiles, the vulnerable parts that protectors try to eliminate because they carry uncomfortable feelings: shame, guilt, and other negative self-referential convictions, fears, or bodily anguish. In Stage One (discussed in Chapter 10), we used IFS techniques to adapt the "response prevention" component of conventional ERP treatment, with the goal of helping clients with OCD transform their relationships with the protectors guarding their OC subsystems. We will continue to engage with protectors in Stage Three.

This chapter, which discusses Stage Two of Self-led ERP, uses the healing steps of IFS therapy to adapt conventional ERP's techniques of exposure, with the goal of creating a similar encounter with exiles. It begins with a reconciliation of these two therapeutic processes—the healing steps of IFS and the exposure step of ERP. Although the two methods are dissimilar on the surface, their shared fundamental goal—an experiential acceptance of feelings that were believed to be intolerable—leads them to a similar result. This chapter then describes the three steps of Stage Two: encountering,

DOI: 10.4324/9781003449812-16

retrieval, and unburdening. Step by step, we follow the case examples of Jason, Aracelli, and Scott to illustrate the steps of an encounter with an exile.

Encountering an Exile *is* Exposure

Exiles in OCD have convictions about fearful or shameful possibilities, or uncertainties about them, or both. They have come to believe and feel that either there is, or there *might* be, something fundamentally wrong with them. They may fear being flawed, negligent, unlovable, or disgusting (shame); selfish, reckless, insensitive, at fault, or amoral (guilt); or defenseless and vulnerable to being—or their loved ones being—physically or mentally harmed (fragile or permeable). These parts have been both terrorized by well-meaning protectors and superficially soothed by them, but what they crave most is the acknowledgement and compassion of Self.

All of us have exiles, pain, and even intrusive thoughts about horrifying things that are the opposite of what we want; people with OCD have parts that engage with those thoughts and interpret them differently. These parts may be responding to brain circuitry that includes a heightened state of alert, a low threshold for alert signaling, and a constant repetition of these alerts. Even when exiles' burdens are released through therapy, the neurobiology underlying OCD may not have changed, so the obsessions repeatedly recur—and this is the reason we may need to return to individual exiles, as well as provide extra help for their protectors, as therapy progresses. Once we help the OC subsystem rely more on Self than on the OC protectors, the exiles can be relieved from their roles as the scapegoat or the receptacle for feared possibilities about identity in the subsystem.

The foundation of first-line OCD treatment is exposure, which is commonly defined as deliberately moving toward previously avoided or anxiety-provoking experiences with an open-minded intention to learn something new. Two notable features of Stage Two of Self-led ERP make it a particularly effective counterpart to conventional exposure-based OCD treatment. First, the way we engage with parts in IFS is to turn toward them with compassion. When the part is an exile, this involves moving toward a previously avoided internal experience in a *Self-led way*—with openness and curiosity. The principles are the same. As acceptance and commitment therapy therapists point out, it's the quality of the contact with the triggering situation that makes exposure effective, and IFS therapy's focus on the presence of Self creates an even more powerful connection. This is the second valuable feature of Self-led ERP. It is highly attuned to other parts in the system as they begin to interfere or mediate the connection between Self and an exiled part. This attunement facilitates the client's ability to stay in close contact with the previously avoided experience—being with the exile. In conventional ERP, as clients sit with their anxieties, no specified method exists for assessing how present or Self-led they are as they sit with the anxiety. The typical exposure process coaches clients not to distract or soothe themselves with grounding techniques, mental compulsions, self-reassurance, or plans to remediate later, but it doesn't necessarily focus on helping clients access Self. This unacknowledged presence or absence of Self may be one factor that influences why clients react unpredictably to exposures.

With IFS we are able to notice compulsive firefighters when they come up as well as other parts that typically interfere. If the client is highly blended with a distressed part during an exposure, learning won't be as robust. When exposures are done from a compliant part, or one who is determined to tough it out rather than lead from Self, clients may lack a certain integrated resilience that helps them maintain their gains going forward. For instance, during therapy a hard-working part makes sure they're doing their best to perform exposure tasks as instructed and follow through on therapy homework, but when the therapist or treatment setting is no longer in place, a lack of trust in Self and no reliable source of inner guidance makes relapses more likely. Or when critical parts continue shaming or minimizing other parts, the valuable inhibitory learning and expectancy violation of exposure therapy may not occur at all. Although many skilled exposure therapists are intuitively aware of these hazards, with IFS, we have a powerful tool to augment the effective principle of exposure with a nuanced attunement to parts that deepens the relational aspects of the experience and achieves long-term healing.

A notable difference with OC systems is the understanding that healing a given exile in an OC subsystem may not have the same immediate impact on its OC protectors as the healing steps generally do in systems where traumas, not OCD, are the driving issue. While it's true that unburdening any exile makes more space for Self, thereby creating a calmer, more curious, internal atmosphere, it is generally *not* the exiles who maintain OCD—no matter how horrible their burdens. OCD resides primarily in the protective parts' interpretation of thoughts and feelings and the actions they take in response. Obsessions and compulsions can continue to make associations that can prompt vulnerable parts to pick up their burdens again. We have to keep in mind that although we are engaging in a healing process with a specific vulnerable part, helping that part alone may not substantially impact the OC subsystem even if we are mindful to involve protectors. It will take a relationship with protectors—the IFS version of response prevention—and typically some ongoing practice (Stage Three) to offer proof that Self can take charge and the protectors can settle down, a result that will fundamentally relieve the OC subsystem itself.

The alarms sounded by obsessional managers point to the core fears, or the burdens of exiles, and represent the shared concern of the OC subsystem as a whole: Obsessional managers generate them, direct them at exiles, and recruit firefighters to extinguish them. Many OC protectors are hugely relieved by the healing steps with an exile; those who are still not able to relax may need more experiences to solidify their ability to trust what they are learning. Sometimes exiles' wounds are the trauma that sets OCD in motion; sometimes OCD predates a distressing event, then latches onto it in an obsessive, hyperfocused way—returning to it repeatedly as proof of danger. This can create a situation in which OCD itself an ongoing traumatizing factor. In either case, increasing the space for Self to be in the lead helps both the OC subsystem and the person's whole system. Whatever may have happened in the historical past, the memories and interpretations of that past are malleable. The healing steps of IFS therapy are designed to transform the disturbing meanings through witnessing, rescripting (the "do over"), retrieval, and unburdening. Following this transformation, we invite the unburdened exile to welcome and integrate new or lost qualities (Schwartz & Sweezy, 2020). This leads Self-led ERP into Stage Three where we emphasize the integration and expand on it.

Before We Continue

The process of encountering exiles in Self-led ERP is a move toward what is most feared. Grounded in the foundation of curiosity and willingness established in Stage One, encountering the exile—turning toward and welcoming it—is the Self-led ERP equivalent of exposure. Our goal is not to extinguish or eliminate the distress or uncertainty, but to learn to accept the part who is suffering and relate to it differently in the present moment. In doing so, we help it release some of the negative beliefs and heavy burdens that make it so challenging for the system to experience in the first place, a release that can transform the whole system's experience of the part. Acceptance and inclusion are key. While the idea that we may just have to accept being anxious is understandably distasteful, discovering that accepting the part who has been burdened with anxiety but may also have gifts and resources makes the prospect feel different to clients. IFS facilitates the inclusion of all parts without the client needing to feel resigned to accepting miserable feelings, or fearful of being overwhelmed by them.

As Stage Two unfolds, the Self-led encounter can progress in a number of ways. We may, as in more typical IFS, *go inside* and invite the exile to connect and share its experience; we may, as in traditional ERP, encounter exiles as they appear during an actual *in vivo* exposure. However we proceed, the intention is to approach the part with distressed feelings, inviting protectors to participate by taking a break from their "jobs" and watching Self handle the experience. In this coordinated Self-led encounter, the client can experience contact with an exile with genuine compassion, acceptance, and empathy while protectors learn to stand down.

As explained in Chapter 2, IFS therapy includes six healing steps: Witnessing, Do Over, Retrieval, Unburdening, Invitation, and Integration (Schwartz & Sweezy, 2020). As I've adapted these healing steps for Self-led ERP, I've focused on the steps most analogous to the exposure process in ERP and saved the last two for Stage Three, when we utilize them to assist in the generalization of the healing experience. The steps follow the arc of an exposure in which a client becomes fully aware of the distress (Witnessing and Do Over), engages differently with the experience (Retrieval), and then allows that experience to be transformed (Unburdening).

Stage Two: Encountering and Unburdening Exiles

Step 1: Witnessing and Do Over.
Step 2: Retrieval.
Step 3: Unburdening and Invitation.

Self-led ERP offers a vast and highly personalized array of prompts during encounters with exiles to help a client maintain compulsion-free contact with the experience. For example, if at any point we notice a client's posture or facial expressions change, or for other reasons suspect another part might have shown up, we can ask about what's happening inside. If our observation was correct and the client says something that indicates a soothing part, a blocking part, or a striving part has entered awareness, we have the client acknowledge that part to see if it will unblend. For instance, someone might say, "I know no one thinks this about me." We could then ask the reassuring part to step back. If it won't, we work with it until it does and then return our attention to the exile. After we do this a few times, clients usually begin to self-report when another part shows up, or when something's happening that needs our attention. Because we expect that protectors often show up during the interaction with the exiles, we are prepared to acknowledge them but also firmly ask them not to interfere. Throughout the healing steps, we continue to check that Self is present enough with the exile that the experience remains one of releasing and learning. Each time we respectfully help the protectors to relax, we help create a little more space for Self.

Step 1: Witnessing and Do Over

The point of the process of encountering exiles in Self-led ERP is to help a client have two general types of new experiences. The first is that of a compassionate Self being fully present with the exiled part, willing to witness its suffering and uncertainty without fixing or judging it. The second is the integrative connection between the Self in the present reality and the exiled part living in a different world, alone with its fears. These two distinct experiences help the client experience external situations that would ordinarily trigger the exile as separate and safe.

Encountering the exiled part is a process that's experiential, relational, and dynamic. These qualities greatly increase our range of options during exposure and help us tailor our interactions to the specific person in front of us, and to that person's individual OC subsystem. We are always mindful of addressing the needs of all the parts in this relational network, so the process can unfold as the parts wish and need. By helping the client to recontextualize the experiences that OCD emerged to avoid, we create a more intimate connection with the experience and a more full-bodied learning experience—deepening exposure in a way that is not usually (or even often) experienced with traditional exposure therapy. This personalization of therapy allows quite a bit of variability in the order of individual steps, and the time we take within each of them.

Witnessing

Witnessing in the context of OCD is the process of willingly sitting with the part who has been exiled by OC protectors—allowing it to share the painful experiences, feelings, and beliefs at the root of its distress and uncertainty. With the permission of protective parts, we turn toward the exile that the OC subsystem has been pushing away for so long. Witnessing requires the OC protectors to willingly pause and allow Self to take the lead as it orchestrates a connection with an exile. In practical terms, creating the conditions for this connection may involve making a literal move toward an external situation that we expect to activate the OC subsystem, such as touching a contaminated object, a move that's typical in conventional exposure therapy. Or we may, instead, make an internal move toward the exile through more purely IFS methods such as *going inside*. For instance, we would suggest the client focus inside, noticing the part that was the subject of protector fears or the part that arises if they imagine the triggering situation. We continue to help the parts that come up to step aside for a fuller experience. Supporting the client's courage, I often ask how it would be to welcome this part with an open heart. Sometimes I still hear protectors grumble in the background; other times the mini-exposures in Stage

One provided enough trust that there's a more immediate sense of relief. The goal is to help the client open to whatever is arising while remaining connected to the calm, confident compassion of Self.

This type of encounter with challenging feelings takes exposure beyond the concept of just staying with it until it habituates. IFS acknowledges that feelings want to be felt, and that they will continue to do whatever it takes to be attended to in the way that they need. To be witnessed is to be seen, heard, felt, and acknowledged. In other words, in this moment of contact, the exiled part is—finally—not alone. Paying attention to exiles in this way is a kind and respectful approach: nurturing the confidence and self-efficacy that enables great Self-leadership with other parts as they come up.

We check for Self-leadership frequently to be sure that the system is not overwhelmed as the exile shares its experience. Sometimes clients get to know exiles primarily through amorphous feelings of fear, dread, or overwhelming uncertainty; just as often, exiles show up with memories from the past that they want to share. What matters is that in this time, in this encounter, Self is present and paying kind attention, inviting and allowing the exiled part to share while also ensuring that protectors are on board.

Do Over

While spending time being compassionately present with and witnessing the exile's experience, the client may remember an early time in life in which caregivers lacked attunement or situations that were traumatic in some way. In those cases, we can offer a "do over," an experience in which the client's Self joins the part in the scene from the past and helps the exile have a new and different experience. This rescripting process is especially helpful in therapy with OC exiles because it is one way for the Self-led client to learn that a previously exiled part can feel accepted without judgment, aversion, or fear and discover that it has the support that it needs. Beginning to forge a trusted connection between the exile in the past and the current reality that Self is available allows the big feelings of exiles to be included and held compassionately, without parts trying to eliminate them. When the painful scene, with all of its distressing emotion, has been fully witnessed and then reexperienced in this new way, clients' experience of internal pain shifts and they're able to relate to it differently. While this may seem to OCD specialists to be a distraction that could potentially undermine the exposure, my experience is that it enhances the intensity and the relevance of the feared feeling, contextualizing it and making the experience of exposures more meaningful. For some clients, a "do over" can enhance the motivation to do exposures; for others, it deepens the experience.

Witnessing and Do over with Aracelli

Aracelli, for instance, had a horror of feeling responsible for harm coming to her family, particularly in situations where she felt she might have been able to prevent it. To help her connect with the exile who felt terrified of being helpless, we first invited her protectors to give their input about how much they were willing to let her experience. At first, understandably, her protectors said they would be overwhelmed by worst-case scenarios. Aracelli began by imagining her son eating a cafeteria lunch that she didn't prepare. As she imagined that scene, all her usual OC parts showed up. First, her Bossy Mom part scolded her and warned that he could choke or get sick, then her terrified exile flared up sparking firefighters who wanted to reassure. Because we had already developed a relationship with her protectors in Stage One, Aracelli could ask them to pause, trust her, and not interfere. Soon she began to feel the dread of not knowing what would happen, and the fear that she had been irresponsible and harmed her child.

As Aracelli considered that she couldn't be certain of his safety and focused on what was coming up inside of her instead of spinning around in the content of the scene, she noticed a feeling of terror and helplessness. When she was able to stay present with that feeling, I asked her how old she felt. She spontaneously began to remember times when she was young and helpless. The memories evoked compassion for that younger version of herself as she was able to witness, from a safe distance, some of what she had gone through and to feel with increasing intensity what that was like. I encouraged her to stay with the part and its feelings as she allowed the memories to play them themselves out, and to continue to send all the compassion that she was noticing to the young part of herself. Being present with the exiled part transformed its experience.

Therapist: How is it for that young part of you to feel your presence and not be alone right now?

Aracelli: It's like she can breathe. She seems surprised that I'm not yelling at her. *[The exile recognizes Self, and notices a different relationship than she's had with the OC protectors.]*

Therapist: Be with her now in the way she needed someone back then but didn't get.

Aracelli: She still feels scared, but it is OK to be scared now that I'm here too.

Here, what's important is that Aracelli is offering a Self-led, secure connection with a young terrified part, which is fundamentally different than the obsessive and compulsive assistance this part has received in the past. Self is helping this part not by remediating its current concerns, but rather by bringing the courage and confidence and the perspective of Self into the experience with the part. With a Self-to-part relationship securely in place, when a triggering situation occurs the part has more moderate feelings because they occur in the context of Self-acceptance. Meal prep time no longer makes Aracelli feel like a scared child. When the time is right, we can offer a retrieval process.

Witnessing and Do over with Scott

Scott had been experiencing disturbing intrusive thoughts about his integrity and intentions. The part that bombarded him with *what ifs* had said it was trying to keep him from being a horrible person. Sometimes he would realize he had been rationalizing and repeating things for hours in order to keep the sinking feeling of uncertainty away. After getting to know the protective parts in Stage One, Scott could feel some spaciousness inside, so I asked, "Would it be OK to give that sinking feeling some attention?" Scott nodded, and I could see his body slump and his head tilt downward as he said, "I could never live with myself if I was that horrible." So, I directed his attention toward the felt sense of that part in his body.

Therapist: Where do you notice the sinking feeling?
Scott: It's in my chest, all the way down into my stomach and back up.
Therapist: Is it OK to stay with the feeling right now and just notice its details, its qualities?
Scott: Yeah, it's both heavy and moving around.
Therapist: Are you open to getting to know it?
Scott: Yes.
Therapist: Ask it what it wants you to know.
Scott: It's reminding me of being little and getting yelled at by my dad and being so confused about why. This is a feeling of not knowing why I feel so bad.

Scott recounted stories of his childhood as they came to mind. Self was there to witness how painful and confusing life had been for the boy. Scott compassionately and calmly listened and helped the young part of himself feel the sense of security and connection that he had needed then. At times during this process, parts would want to explain or interpret, but each time a protector came in we gently asked it to not interfere. In other moments, Scott felt nearly overcome by the shameful feelings carried by that part, which had come to believe it was truly bad. But as we sat with the part, Scott was able to be with it and was amazed by the feeling that he could stay there without the ritualizing parts coming to the rescue. It may seem that the memories from that past could function as distractions, but in the process of IFS they often intensify the feeling that the OC and other parts were exiling. The only shift is that clients report that it feels more deep or more intimate than in regular ERP. In my experience, the feared experience is held in awareness throughout.

Since uncertainty, shameful self-referential beliefs (*I am a monster*), and the embodied feelings of fear seemed so real to Scott (as they do to so many with OCD), the prospect was initially threatening to his protectors, who—without enough access to a trustworthy Self—wanted to step back in. Parts may be afraid of the exile or afraid of the whirlwind of rituals that compulsive firefighters have engaged in previously. With experience and the supportive Self of the therapist lending confidence and calm, protectors become increasingly willing to allow Self to be with the part, eventually revealing those beliefs and feelings to be false narratives, or burdens that the vulnerable parts took on and therefore can let go of.

Traditionally an exposure therapist would encourage the client to lean into the anxiety while refraining from engaging in any distracting conversation or other self-soothing or grounding activities. Sometimes this leaves the client toughing it out on the outside but regulating anxiety internally with the silent assistance of reassuring voices inside. In such an exposure, Scott might have reassured himself throughout, without even realizing that he was doing it, let alone understanding that he was not fully engaging with the exposure—instead reinforcing a reliance on firefighters in dealing with the big feelings of exiles. Because IFS therapists know that Self can be with intense feelings without being harmed, we regularly check for Self by asking, "How do you feel toward the part?" If the answer is less than kind, we help the client unblend from protectors who may have jumped in.

ERP therapists know that allowing the fear to surface and be fully experienced without grounding or using other relaxation techniques can create a powerful learning experience, which is at the core of the healing in OCD treatment. With Self-led ERP protectors become willing (even if begrudgingly or cautiously so) to step back, and Self is naturally open and curious, able to connect with the exiled part and witness whatever comes up (strong feelings, fears, memories, stories). By witnessing from Self while continuing to help protector parts relax, Self-led ERP similarly facilitates a powerful learning. Clients stay with the experience of exiled anxiety, discomfort, disgust, or uncertainty, welcoming them with compassion for an extended period of time, becoming more comfortable with the feelings while also learning that they can handle the experience. Rather than dismissing, negating, or even transcending painful feelings, real healing comes when we relate to them with tenderness and respect.

Witnessing and Do over with Justin

When the protectors have stepped back and we suggest turning toward the part or the feelings they have been protecting against, many clients—like

Aracelli and Scott—encounter a part who is experienced as a younger version of themselves, but others do not. For Justin, the exiled part showed up as a ball of energy that he reported he felt all over his body, and that threatened to take over. Establishing a comfortable distance from that ball of energy, we continued to help all parts who showed up with reactions to the exile. With Self in the leadership role, Justin could experience the part. As he let it register and respond to the new experience of being welcomed, rather than extinguished, it gradually shifted, first in size then in color. Finally, it became a wave that Justin knew he could attend to with compassion. This shift occurred because parts of Justin who feared it or wanted it gone—as well as any parts of the therapist who might have felt that a grounding or relaxation tool was warranted—stepped back in favor of allowing Justin to open to the part and all that came with it.

Step 2. Retrieval

Very often exiled parts are described as being in a different world and with OCD this is true as well. Inference-based cognitive behavioral therapy theorists coined a term, the "OCD Bubble" (O'Connor & Aardema, 2013) to describe an internal mindset in which different rules apply, and every possible imaginary horror takes on a gruesome likelihood. In IFS this inner world is often but not always connected to a wounding past. Either way, after an emotionally corrective experience in which an exile feels attended to, the client's experience of that imagined world, or that other time and place begins to shift. Retrieval is the healing step in which we offer a change of venue. Through this new connection with Self, exiles discover that they can move into the present as a part of the client's whole internal system. When that happens, the Self is able to bring the exiled part into present reality and can invite it into more harmonious and welcoming and reality focused relationships with the other parts of the client's larger system.

When blended with an OC part, a person can become highly absorbed in the imaginal world to such an extent that it feels possible that a tiny speck of dirt can spread like wet paint to an entire house or that years later an object can still be contaminated. In the inner OC universe, a bad thought feels like it could result in a family member being harmed, and using scissors too quickly feels like it could mean one might be a serial killer. When the parts that hold these fears are introduced to the Self, they can emerge from this inner world or the OCD bubble into the client's current reality—whether they are protectors or exiles. Rather than the person seeing the world through the eyes of a part lost in strange and scary world, the part can opt to see the real world through the eyes of the Self in the here and now. An update occurs when the part is retrieved. The process can be surprisingly natural and simple, and here in Stage Two it is facilitated by having the client simply ask the exile if it would like to leave the time and place where it is stuck.

Retrieval with Aracelli

Therapist: Would she like to stay where she is or be somewhere else?
Aracelli: She clearly does not want to be where she is.
Therapist: Let her know she can be anywhere she wants.
Aracelli: All of a sudden I'm seeing us in my own house instead of where I lived as a kid. *[Now she will be able to shift the nature of her relationship with this part.]*

With the OC subsystem, we do need to be careful. Retrieval may be affected by OC protectors' fears, so we draw on the creative nature of Self to find a solution. With OCD, I have noticed that protective parts sometimes object to a retrieval because they are afraid that the exile is contaminated—especially before unburdening—and want the exile to unburden in the past and only then come into the present. All that is fine, as long as the client's Self agrees. Be sure to trust and follow the needs of the client's system, and when retrieval is called for (it's not needed by every part), understand that bringing the exile into the present world of the client may happen in small increments over time.

Retrieval with Justin

At first, Justin's OC protectors had fears about the idea of bringing the exiled part into their world because they were not yet certain that wouldn't contaminate everything. One firefighter wanted to help the part "unburden" before coming into the present—which sounded eerily similar to decontamination compulsions in which family members are asked to take shoes or even clothes off before entering the house. I inquired and it was immediately clear that it was a part making the request, and that is was a compulsion. In time, that part was open to a compromise, and the ball of energy could be experienced in the present, just as it was, because its burdens could be seen as fears, not realities.

Step 3: Unburdening and Invitation

Once their predicament—their uncertainty, anxiety, shame, guilt, worthlessness, or vulnerability—has been compassionately encountered, and they've become securely connected with Self, exiled parts are helped to release their stuck beliefs through unburdening. By gaining new connections with Self, exiles also gain a different way to experience old burdens; no longer must they rely only on their OC protectors for help. What follows is highly varied. For some parts, it's a cathartic experience of letting go of old beliefs; these parts unburden quickly. For others, burdens may fall away in stages, as they gain more and more connection to Self. If an exile is ready to let go of the negative messages that it has been stuck with, we facilitate that. If not, we help the part manage its burdens in other ways, such as suggesting it place them in storage, or even just set them down for the time being. When the exile is ready, we facilitate the process of letting go, supporting the protective parts in allowing it to happen.

When parts become burdened, they begin to believe negative messages about themselves or the world around them. With OCD, exiles are often burdened by uncertainty and concern about what might be true. This necessarily displaces some of the innocence, openness, and sensitivity they may have had. The unburdening of old beliefs creates space to invite back strengths, qualities, and capacities that may have been sidelined or lost. We conclude by asking exiles to invite back qualities that they needed, wanted, or had lost as a result of being burdened, and to appreciate all parts for showing up and participating.

Unburdening and Invitation with Aracelli

After the terrified, guilt-ridden part that was a four-year-old girl grew to feel safe sitting with Aracelli in the present, I asked Aracelli to see if the part still carried burdens. It's often surprising how clearly clients' parts can identify and articulate these stuck feelings; often they're lodged in specific spaces within their bodies and have a palpable presence of some sort, showing up as pressure, tightness, heaviness, or terror.

Therapist: Does the little girl still carry other burdens, or negative beliefs about herself from the past?
Aracelli: She does. She feels them like lead sitting in her solar plexus.
Therapist: Ask her if there's anything she wants to say about the lead or if she's ready to let it go.
Aracelli: She wants it gone. How does she let it go?
Therapist: She can do whatever she wants. She can bury it or let it go up into the atmosphere or into the ocean or do whatever feels right to her.
Aracelli: OK. It's gone. And now she's smiling at me. She feels like a child ought to feel, free and light.

Because Aracelli's Self was no longer blocked from sitting with her young part, who had been filled with terror, that part felt permission to have and express her fear within the safety of the new relationship. And because her protectors had been persuaded to stop pushing the formerly exiled part away, the intensity of the fear began to dissipate. As Aracelli's relationship with the part became one of acceptance and compassion, the young girl no longer felt alone with the fear, and the protectors no longer felt it was their job alone to eliminate it. The parts were all still there but their relationships with one another had been transformed.

While the goal of most approaches to exposure therapy is to change *behavior*, the goal of Stage Two of Self-led ERP is to change the internal *relationships* that drive the unwanted behavior: in this case, a repeating loop that reinforces protector activities that only add to burdens. For Aracelli, her loops of alerting and reassuring kept a young part of her burdened by fear. Now that she knows and has integrated her young part when it becomes activated, Aracelli's Self can be with the feelings, and the part no longer has to deal with them alone. Now that Aracelli's part has learned to trust Self, Aracelli can experience the potentially frightening stimuli of imperfection and uncertainty as acceptable. The next time her son wants to eat at a friend's house, she can welcome the fear as a young part of herself who needs her love. She can turn toward this part, who now elicits compassion instead of reactivity, and help it settle with the help and guidance of Self-leadership. The parts of her who interact around anxiety-evoking situations can now do so harmoniously and with balance as a result of Self being in the lead. Having gained some understanding and compassion for the part of her who felt that she was in danger if she made a mistake, Aracelli noticed a new connection to the inquisitive, curious aspects of herself she'd lost, along with the creativity that they had fueled, and she was able to commit to staying in touch with those qualities going forward.

Unburdening with Scott

Once Scott was able to update his system and show his parts the world as he saw it in the present, there was a palpable shift. The young part, once vulnerable to his father shaming, could look to Scott to feel secure rather than seek the safety offered by compulsive firefighters. When we asked the boy if he had taken on any negative beliefs about himself, he named several. He believed thinking a bad thought was as bad as acting on it, that he was either all good or all bad. When he felt accepted by Scott's kindness and concern, he said he could let those beliefs fall away.

Encountering exiles with enough Self-energy, clients also develop greater awareness of the experience of being blended with OC parts. It becomes easier to notice the moment when they cross over from a state of Self-leadership, in which they are in touch with reality, to an internal world, where imaginal absorption increases OCD doubts and moves them further away from calm. They can begin to feel it when they enter the OC subsystem bubble. With access to Self the client discovers that OCD makes them less secure, even though it seems to be about safety-seeking. They see that the efforts of firefighters doing compulsions to try to resolve obsessional managers' doubts and fears only increase the stress and anguish of the OC subsystem. Learning to access an imaginal world, to facilitate bringing stuck parts out of their place in that internal OC bubble, is a powerful shift. It strengthens clients' ability to function in a manner that is grounded in the clarity of Self-leadership and the reality of the senses. They become confident that they can be with distress and uncertainty and that it is meaningful and healing to do so.

Moving onto Stage Three

Unburdening, the final step of Stage Two of Self-led ERP, can lead right into Stage Three. When exiles feel seen and heard they relax and—as anyone would—they feel less invested in making sure everyone can feel, hear, and understand their pain. Having been acknowledged, they settle a bit and then are in a better position to release the feelings and beliefs that drive the OC subsystem. But completing this step can also signal a return to Stage One if protectors have not accepted Self's leadership and are silently still doing their jobs until they are able to jump back in. By taking the time to check in with a client's OC protectors and inviting them, again, to be a part of the process, we learn their status and, responding appropriately, minimize the occurrence of backlash later on.

When we re-envision exposure in this way, offering a Self-led encounter with an exile who feels fully welcomed and understood, clients often report a feeling of having gotten to know a part of themselves with an intimacy they'd never before experienced. Actual learning has happened because they were able to get to know their fearful parts while maintaining differentiation, so that their compulsive parts didn't feel the need to come rushing in and put a stop to the experience.

Typically, IFS therapy doesn't include explicit post-unburdening steps, and such steps will not always be necessary in Self-led ERP. But in my experience, many people with OCD need additional support and practice to solidify the new experiences that the parts have had together and to build trust in Self-leadership. Obsessional managers often continue to send disturbing alarm messages, which can create new burdens or cause exiles to pick up their old burdens unless the real nature of the OC protectors is made clear: They are parts, not Self, but they are used to running the show. That's why it's so essential for people with OCD to consolidate their experiential learning—with continued support—by taking these new internal relationships out into the real world and practicing trying something different. When they successfully engage in life and have meaningful values-driven experiences, OC protectors slowly begin to accept that Self-leadership is not only possible but also preferable. A new homeostasis can begin to develop as they relax their control of life situations.

References

Nicely, S. (2018). *Is Fred in the refrigerator? Taming OCD and reclaiming my life*. Nicely Done, LLC.

O'Connor, K., & Aardema, F. (2013). *Clinician's handbook for obsessive-compulsive disorder: Inference-based therapy*. Wiley-Blackwell.

Schwartz, R. C., & Sweezy, M. (2020). *Internal family systems therapy* (2nd ed.). The Guilford Press.

Chapter 12

Stage Three
Reconnecting with Protectors

Stage One of Self-led ERP, my reframing of exposure and response prevention therapy (Chapter 10) presented an Internal Family Systems (IFS) lens on several key principles of OCD treatment: (1) normalizing intrusive thoughts as the work of obsessional managers, (2) facilitating disengagement from these obsessional parts through unblending, and (3) reducing the over-responsibility of OC parts dedicated to keeping the whole system calm and safe. Through incremental experiments that foster security by relying instead on Self, these OC protectors become more willing to dial down—or at least pause—their safety-seeking efforts, learning to trust that Self-leadership provides some hope of a better way. Stage Two of treatment (Chapter 11), grounded in the acceptance of uncertainty, demonstrated how exiled parts, with the compassionate, clear-seeing presence of Self, can be witnessed and welcomed even as OC protectors stand by, watch, and learn that their interventions are not required. Now, with greater capacity to differentiate parts from Self, the feelings of dread, doom, and danger that are so common in OCD can be faced with more stability.

Sometimes unburdening exiles is enough to convince even OC protectors to let go of their extreme positions. But obsessive-compulsive disorder (OCD) is generally perpetuated less by a traumatized part, that is, the burdens of exiles, than by the insistence of obsessional managers on the primacy of their doubts and the stories by which they elaborate potential dire consequences. So, with OCD, it's more likely that an additional stage of purposeful reengagement with the protective system will be required to help OC protectors relax. That's what Stage Three of Self-led ERP is designed to address. Returning our focus to the OC protectors, we concentrate on facing feared situations without compulsive firefighters jumping in, helping them to recognize Self-leadership by taking the transformative internal experience of Stages One and Two out into the world.

We navigate Stage Three by integrating the changes that have occurred through relationship building and practice. The internal shifts involve updating the system and helping the obsessional managers to let go of

DOI: 10.4324/9781003449812-17

their heightened sense of responsibility and the other burdens that drive the process of obsessional behaviors (Steps 1 and 2). Then all parts rehearse new options, allowing the whole system to practice new trust, and confidence-building experiences (Step 3), as we facilitate an integration of what has been learned to foster the balance and harmony that grows with Self-leadership (Step 4).

This chapter begins with the rationale and need for an additional stage with OC subsystems, then offers specific steps and tools based on the patterns of protective parts rather than exiles. With these options in place, this chapter describes the steps of Stage Three, illustrated with examples and transcripts from the case material we've been following.

Why We Need Stage Three with OCD

Sometimes, after the healing steps with an exile, protectors are still not interested in letting go of their extreme positions. That's the exception to the rule in typical IFS treatment, occurring when there are legacy burdens to address, unburdening was incomplete, backlash occurred, or a new issue intervenes (Anderson et al., 2017). In the treatment of OCD, however, it's common: Exposures are not a one and done experience, and there are often additional burdens in the protective system. While the identity burdens of exiles may provide the thematic material for obsessional managers, exiles are not usually the cause or driving force that perpetuates OCD. Their unburdening will create a shift, and more access to Self, but it is only the beginning. That's why IFS for OCD adds a third stage of Self-led ERP, designed to anticipate what we might otherwise think of as an unexpectedly challenging protective subsystem. When OC protectors continue to do their jobs even once exiles are retrieved or seem relieved, we understand it to be an ordinary stage of the work.

Clients with OCD often report that even after healing work with an exile, their obsessional managers say things like, "This is just what I do," and that the protective behavior continues to feel like a habit, ingrained and hard to break, or that their protectors seem to be operating on autopilot, continuing with their work as if nothing has changed. From an IFS perspective, we suspect that they are still motivated by something, even though they seem less clear on what that might be. Other times it seems that because the previous homeostasis of the OC subsystem has been shifted by the retrieval of an exile, the protectors may feel territorial and concerned about losing their jobs. Many factors can play a role, and with OCD often the physiology of the sticky brain circuitry is one of them. Although exiles and their burdens may continue to threaten instability for a variety of reasons, those concerns would bring us back into Stage Two.

Stage Three is designed to demonstrate to the protectors that with Self-leadership, the exile, even for all of its strong feelings of anxiety, shame, or uncertainty, is not the actual problem. Rather, the struggle lies with the outsized efforts of OC protectors to prevent or eliminate potential distress. Still, welcoming the exile can take some time, and some clients worry when OC protectors keep going. For instance, when clients with OCD discover that sitting with uncertainty about having caused harm, or fear of getting sick, is tolerable or not as difficult as they expected, they usually experience palpable relief. So, if or when obsessions continue, clients can experience confusion about how to proceed. Some approaches, acceptance and commitment therapy (ACT), for instance, suggest noting obsessions and then letting them go (Hayes et al., 2003), allowing them to flow by like the chyron at the bottom of a news screen. Inference-based cognitive behavioral therapy (I-CBT) focuses on reality sensing to help the client redirect attention out of the inner world of the OCD bubble into the external five senses and common sense reality (O'Connor & Aardema, 2013). Self-led ERP can do both. We help protectors let go of their extreme (and no longer functional) beliefs and we help the protectors practice living in a system in which the formerly exiled part is included and welcomed. These new relationships foster greater Self-leadership in even the most rambunctious, noisy, and demanding of protective systems.

OC protectors that don't adjust easily to this reorganization may have burdens of their own in the form of beliefs about the world or their responsibilities, fears about losing control, and the overblown ramifications and risks they foresee. These burdens, as well as the protectors' own natures, can continue to drive their behavior and continue to affect both the OC subsystem and the whole system. I often see OC protectors who want to "be sure" the unburdening is "100% complete" or who want to go through the process again because it offered relief. These behaviors indicate that the parts are not motivated solely by an intolerance of the anxiety, shame, or distress of the exile but by their own doubts, interpretations, and inferences of possibilities. Obsessional managers may also have inherited genetic or family legacy burdens that drive their doubts and their difficulty accepting exiles. Compulsive firefighters responding to the intractability of obsessions may still feel they serve an important purpose. These obsessional parts function in idiosyncratic ways that depend on many factors, including the type of OCD, age of onset, severity, structural issues, and the particular neural pathways impacted.

With OCD it is best to balance the internal, relational aspects of IFS with the external action-oriented moves from the more behavioral approaches. If clients are open to a more experiential and experimental approach, ideally, we move from Step 1 directly to Step 3 and engage with more of the valued activities of life, helping protectors learn from experience. If this is not feasible or appropriate for some reason, we move to Step 2 in which we help protectors unburden using a more typical IFS approach.

> **Stage Three: Reconnecting with Protectors**
>
> Step 1. Update.
> Step 2. Going inside.
> Step 3. Going outside.
> Step 4. Bringing it all together.

Step 1: Update

We begin the first step of Stage Three by updating the OC protective subsystem to begin the process of integrating the new learning from Stages One and Two. We explore protectors' willingness to recognize Self and establish whether they are ready to let go of their extreme roles. If they're not yet willing to relinquish extreme positions, we explore why not and assist with unblending and unburdening as needed to help clients become increasingly able to identify and unhook from the narratives that stir up the OC subsystem.

Our intentional return to OC protectors after we've engaged in the healing work with exiles helps the protectors find new roles or more balanced approaches to their old jobs. OC protectors often hold out until they can see Self in action. They need the presence of Self to heal their own wounds so that they can let go of their belief that they need to be sure—100% sure—that their particular concern will never occur.

We begin by looking for some clarity about how the OC protectors responded to the encounter with the exile. Again, some protectors may relax right away, as we'll see with Scott. Some may not be aware of our work with the exile or may not believe it matters, and so will need to engage in life activities before seeing that they don't need to continue to incessantly sound such loud alarms. This was the case with Aracelli. Others may have burdens of their own or additional exiles that they are trying to keep at bay, as happened with Justin. These are not the only possibilities, but they are common and serve as a way to illustrate the range of protector reactions that Stage Three is intended to address.

Have Protectors Relaxed?

As we have seen, a Self-led encounter with an exiled part carrying negative beliefs and strong emotions is an IFS version of internal exposure: The client turns toward a challenging feeling with openness, and in so doing, the feeling is encountered and transformed. Since exposure is known to work for OCD, it makes sense that a fully experienced encounter with an exile will sometimes be all that's needed to help the OC subsystem: The obsessional manager develops trust and stops sounding unnecessary alarms; the compulsive firefighter no longer needs to jump in; and the subsystem becomes far less reactive even if some trepidation remains.

Self-led ERP often unfolds just as in this scenario—especially when the OC subsystem is mild or newly developed. The next time I saw Scott, for instance, he was relieved: Encountering his exiles with compassion allowed these parts of him to be felt. Once that happened fully, the parts were no longer as threatening to his scrupulous protectors. They had experienced and could trust that Scott's Self was able to handle the powerful "sinking" feelings of uncertainty and shame carried by the exile and that by accepting and welcoming the formerly scary part, he had helped it to let go of its burdens. At this point Scott's Quality Controller was able to accept him being sure "enough" that he had good intentions. For example, in the following days, Scott was able to turn in an assignment without checking every reference several times. His part that set standards still wanted to know that he had done his best not to plagiarize, and Scott's Self was able to offer enough of a sense of security that the protective part did not start amplifying the worst-case scenario in search of a reassurance compulsion. What this meant for Scott was that he was not plagued by intrusive thoughts all day as usual, and when a thought did pop up, he was able to acknowledge it and let it go. Instead of telling himself, "maybe I cheated, maybe I didn't" as he might be instructed to do in standard OCD treatment, his internal dialogue was more along the lines of Self talking to a part and saying, "let me handle it," as a parent might tell a child worried about adult issues. After checking in and finding these parts significantly calmer, we still progressed through the steps of Stage Three to reinforce the confidence that these parts had begun to develop in Scott's ability to make decisions from Self.

If Not, Why Not?

In contrast, unburdening the exile sometimes seems to have very little effect on OC protectors: they seem unaware of the Self-to-part relationships that have developed, or unimpressed. They continue in their roles as if on autopilot, and will need updates to be reinforced with repetition. It may seem that more needs to be done to help an exile unburden completely or cope with burdens that return. With OCD, however, it is often also the case that the obsessional manager continues to frighten the exile and other parts when it fires off its doubts for no apparent reason. Most often, we find that OC protectors are burdened or simply need more help to stop perpetuating the cycle—especially when they are responding to neurobiology. If an anxiety signal flares up, and protectors respond to that *uh-oh* by sounding alarms, telling stories, and casting blame, exiles may be pushed aside and then be inclined to pick up their recently discarded burdens. It is not uncommon to hear vulnerable parts say the OC protectors are scaring them. When this happens, it's helpful to offer psychoeducation for clients so that they can understand that protective parts in OCD are frequently responding to the brain–body system. The low threshold for firing of alarm circuitry in the brain means that one part or another will jump in to make meaning of the alarm until Self is more accessible. With practice, the secure Self will take on more of that role and mediate these internal experiences.

After Aracelli's breakthroughs welcoming her young, frightened part, I was curious to see what she'd experience in the week between sessions.

Therapist: How'd your week go?
Aracelli: After we helped that young part, I started feeling more calm overall, and it has stuck. But I still have these thoughts and images that just keep coming. I'm just not as flooded with anxiety by them anymore.
Therapist: Those parts are still doing their jobs?
Aracelli: Yeah. It's mainly the bossy one.
Therapist: And you're aware of her being there now?
Aracelli: Yeah, she's just kind of there . . . with a lack of awareness and just keeps showing up without any sense that maybe there's not the same purpose to it anymore or even the same result. She's just kind of on automatic or something . . . showing up and wanting to warn me. "Stay away from" this or that. "Make sure you" this or that!

Realizing that there was more to be done before we understood what her OC subsystem needed, I wondered aloud if Aracelli was curious about the processes driving these obsessional narratives. She was, and so we continued to explore internally.

The energy level and intensity of protectors who don't stop may become milder or stay just as intense as they had been. Protectors keep working for a variety of reasons, and although we may not know the etiology of their persistence, we can ask the part what it thinks is its function, which will give us a place to start. As with Aracelli, Justin had been able to witness and help an exile, and yet he had a protector, the OC protector he called his Scout, who wouldn't give up even as it felt a greater presence of Self. It would take additional exploration to see what might be motivating this part to continue to be so frantic.

Therapist: What are you noticing?
Justin: The Scout is pacing back and forth, yelling at me. He still thinks that he needs to watch out for bad things coming. If I'm unprepared, I could end up in another situation where something could contaminate me and that would be intolerable. *[Because Justin is speaking from a part, we can see that he is blended with a younger part who feels unprepared and vulnerable to contamination.]*
Therapist: How do you feel toward the Scout?
Justin: I'm intimidated by him—
Therapist: Can you let the part who's intimidated know you are here?
Justin: Oh, I see. Yeah, I'm reminding him that I'm here, and he can relax.
Therapist: OK, can you still see the Scout?
Justin: Yes.
Therapist: How do you feel toward him now?
Justin: More concerned for him, I guess. He seems scared. I wonder what it will take for him to relax.
Therapist: How is he responding to you?
Justin: He isn't really responding to me at all . . . He just keeps scanning and pointing things out.
Therapist: Would he like your help?
Justin: He doesn't think I *can* help.
Therapist: Ah. Remind him of who you are, where you live, and what you do now. Let him know what just happened with the exile. *[Updating.]*
Justin: He knows; he just seems unimpressed and keeps pacing. *[The protector needs more proof.]*

If a client's OC protectors have relaxed—as Scott's did—you can move on to Step 3, in which you engage the external world, including the triggers that the client identified during assessment. Because OCD can be severely limiting, therapists using IFS for OCD will usually need to bring the benefits gained from internal work, that is, increased Self-leadership, outside and into the client's lived experience. In other words, we honor the overall good of the whole system, internal and external, as the presiding intention of treatment, and this includes reducing the avoidances that are constraining a person's ability to function. So, as we did in the first stage of treatment, we will want to use engagement with the client's actual triggers as a guide for our interactions with OC parts. If protectors are still objecting, we can help them first by taking a little more time going inside.

Step 2: Going Inside

Keeping in mind that most of our clients with OCD have substantially less freedom than they did before the OC subsystem took over, a primary goal of IFS for OCD is to help them reclaim lost territory through Self-leadership. So, we encourage parts to engage the world outside. However, we also know, from the IFS perspective, that protectors often have their own burdens and when that is the case it is helpful to address those first. Legacy burdens may be driving their behavior or the typical beliefs held by obsessional managers that include a heightened sense of responsibility to ensure safety, a tendency to over-estimate danger and the potential consequences of risk, as well as beliefs about the importance of thoughts that are interpreted as just as dangerous or equal to the action (thought – action fusion).

Obsessional managers believe that catastrophic results will occur if they fail to monitor, warn, and recruit firefighters to prevent exiles from flooding the system. If an exile is burdened with shame, guilt, inadequacy, loss of control, or a sense of impending doom, the corresponding protector is burdened with the beliefs that those feelings would be devastating, could come true at any time, and would create intolerable and interminable damage if they did. Clearly, they think, it's their responsibility to prevent all that from happening. The OC protectors can end up quite frightened and wounded themselves.

Aracelli's Struggles with Her Protectors

Clients will often notice that everyday triggers have become easier to deal with, but the challenging ones remain difficult. In the week since our last session, Aracelli had experimented with lightly acknowledging her protectors while staying Self-led. She was pleased with her new freedom, but unsure of how durable it would be in the face of continual demands.

Therapist: If you are ready to explore this part that sends you warnings let her know you're here.
Aracelli: She doesn't seem to notice me. She's just frantic and keeps repeating "What if" this and "what if" that! *[It's common in OCD for protectors not to notice Self.]*
Therapist: Acknowledge what you see her experiencing and try again to let her know you're here to help.
Aracelli: Now she sees me, and is aware of me, but just nods and keeps on doing what she's doing.
Therapist: How do you respond to that?
Aracelli: Well, I understand, and I'd like to show her that I can handle things.

Stage Three: Reconnecting with Protectors

At this point we have a choice. We might opt to spend some time exploring the motives of this protector, being careful not to engage with the content of the concerns. But since the part seems to be operating without a connection to Aracelli and without other clear concerns, I suspect it's responding to neurological alarms and opt to move on to Step Three and facilitate Aracelli's ability to show this part how it would be to let Self take the lead.

Justin's Protector's Second Job

Often when protectors won't give up, it's not because they're unnecessarily stuck, it's because they're still at work—doing a second job that we haven't yet discovered. After Justin and I were able to unburden the wounded exile we had found, he was frustrated that his obsessions kept coming. Although he was much less reactive, and he was able to stay mostly Self-led instead of getting blended with parts that wanted him to do washing compulsions, Justin continued to be swamped with intrusive thoughts about things being dirty. So, we explored and discovered that his contamination protector was also guarding a second exile—one his protector still considered far too dangerous to accept.

Therapist: Will you ask your Scout why he's still so protective?
Justin: Interesting! He knows that the wounded part is no longer stuck in the scary past *[He means the exile we retrieved and unburdened earlier.]* but he still says he needs to be on guard.
Therapist: Ask him if he'd be willing to let you show him how things can be. *[Updating.]*
Justin: I *am* showing him the things I've done recently and I'm reminding him how much better I've gotten . . . but he's saying that it'll still be awful if he stops.
Therapist: Hmm. See if he wants to say more about that. *[I want to know if something is motivating him.]*
Justin: There's something else that he's trying to keep away—it's like a dark ball of dirtiness.
Therapist: Ask him if he'd like it if we could help that part.
Justin: He says he's not sure, but he seems to be willing to at least let me try.

If the part needing help is another exile, we move back into Stage Two with this new exile so the client can heal that part. Justin and I spent several sessions sitting with this new exiled part, which was carrying vile, disgusting feelings. This time, as Justin's Self got to know the stuck feelings carried by this part, we checked in with his OC protectors to see if they were watching. They were watching closely, and as Justin witnessed the experiences this part chose to share with him, they experienced Justin's Self capably handling the strong sensations and feelings of disgust. Eventually, when the exile finally confessed its shameful belief that it was, in fact, dirty and vile, Justin's compassionate Self embraced the part, and upon being seen fully and accepted and held imaginally, its identification with that shame melted away. The unburdening offered the psychological healing that needed to happen for Justin to be able to access enough Self-energy to calm the OC protectors who were still stirring up his subsystem. This return to the Stage Two encounter with an exile before returning to Stage Three is common with OCD and demonstrates the flexibility that the Self-led ERP approach can bring to OCD treatment.

Sometimes when OC protectors are overly identified with their jobs, and they see the havoc they've created in their own internal and external systems, they take on burdens and are unable or unwilling to change for a variety of reasons. Sometimes it would require them to break a loyalty bond or acknowledge what they'd done. In the process of sounding endless alarms over the course of decades, burdened OC protectors may have lost touch with reality. It can be frightening for them to let go of the belief system that they meticulously developed over time.

Justin's hypervigilent protector, the Scout, seemed aware that Justin had demonstrated that he could be with the uncertainty and the feelings of disgust that his system had so valiantly tried to exile. After further conversation, it became clear that this part believed that to stop meant that it was responsible for the damage to the years of his life that Justin spent unable to function. Realizing that this protector needed Justin to witness how painful its extreme role had been, we focused on helping it release the negative beliefs about itself. These burdens were keeping it attached to doing its job even without the motivation of an exile. Once this protector felt compassionately witnessed it let go of its burdens and could invite in qualities previously experienced as capacities and ultimately relax.

In a subsequent session, Justin remarked that he could now move in and out of feelings of contamination without being overwhelmed by them. He also reported that the Scout was noticing him for the first time. And although Justin was still hearing the Scout's warnings, they were less alarming in everyday situations. This progress suggested to me that we were ready to progress to the next steps of Stage Three, in which his parts could develop experience by engaging in a wider variety of conditions.

Step 3: Going Outside

Once clients have had the experience of Self in the lead as they interact with their most feared possibilities, we need to help their OC protectors find a way to truly absorb and integrate this information. Because learning is experiential, and trust is built through personal experience, we offer protectors an opportunity to try something new and see for themselves how well Self is able to manage. The offering is freedom: the freedom to engage in life with courage, in a way that previously seemed out of reach.

It takes a while to learn that an experience is safe and tolerable once it has been tagged as dangerous. But for change to occur, all parts must have a chance to see each other at work in harmony with Self in the context of the situations that trigger their OCD. We help the client decide which experiences they most value having, and ask their parts not to interfere while they move toward those situations where they're willing to take a little risk. As was the case with Scott after encountering his exile and updating protectors, an individual client may pretty quickly navigate formerly impossible situations without a hitch. Or, as with Aracelli and Justin, the client's OC protectors may need to practice newly learned trust in Self before they can let go of their old strategies. Building these Self-to-part relationships is important and can take time, but once Self is more regularly in the lead, a greater amount of uncertainty is increasingly tolerable for increasing amounts of time.

In this step, we reengage with OC protectors, helping them practice operating within their new, less-extreme positions—and we help interpret the experience and provide evidence of safety to these protectors. This step is often the most critical one in the healing process, and one we revisit again and again because we know that the fact that protectors have relaxed in one area doesn't mean that their behavior will generalize to all areas. Even when exiles are healed and the intensity of their burdens is relieved, and even when protectors have relaxed and their own burdens are healed, a situation that seems too new or too different than one they have determined is safe may cause their behavior to escalate. We help the protectors find a role or job that's both suitable to their nature and valuable within the system as a whole and practice this more moderate approach with the presence of Self even when protectors are dubious. Self guides this process in a trustworthy way, proposing new activities as experiments (exposures) designed collaboratively from within to enhance the harmony and balance of the internal relationships.

Since OCD can limit life to the point of disability, it's important to help our clients actually reengage with the experiences that they have been avoiding. Once Self is more accessible, even OC protectors are willing to try new things and engage in the life events formerly seen as too risky. Courage, one of the 8 C's, involves making the choice to engage in valued activities in the face of fear, discomfort, or uncertainty, knowing that brains may overinflate concerns about risk. The heart of Stage Three is making courageous choices even when OC protectors are not entirely sure they are on board. We ask them to take a risk and give Self a try with the promise of more sustainable long-term relief. Then we proceed to collaborate with them so that they participate in the intrinsic reward.

What we are doing in this step is allowing a client's Self to guide the choices and helping parts who may struggle learn to trust and relax back. We are not changing behavior from a managerial part with an agenda, but with compassion, patience, and perseverance, we highlight the shift in the internal dynamics that drive behaviors. This approach allows Self-leadership to arise and helps the client to rise to the occasion. Leaning on the principle of exposure, Self-led ERP demonstrates that anxiety itself is safe and tolerable and that safety behaviors fail to provide the internal security that can only be found with Self-led experience.

Aracelli's Courageous Choices

Aracelli's parenting had been greatly compromised by her OCD, so when I asked what mattered most to her, she said that she wanted to be able to give her children a reasonable amount of freedom. (In this conversation, we were speaking remotely.)

Therapist: How would it be for your parts to try something new today?
Aracelli: Letting my kids have more freedom is something that matters a lot to me. I would love to let my kids go play at the neighbor's house without me for an afternoon, but I've just always stayed with them so I think it would be really uncomfortable.
Therapist: I hear a part of you that anticipates it being uncomfortable. Is there any part that sees it differently?
Aracelli: Yeah, but trying that right now, that's a big "no way."
Therapist: OK; so is there something that your parts would be willing to let you try?
Aracelli: Yes, actually, my husband came home from the grocery store with pre-cut watermelon yesterday, and I told him that there was no way I could let the kids have that. But maybe that would be nice for them. It's hot out and it looks really good.
Therapist: What if we were to try that right now . . . so that I can be here with you and with any parts that have strong feelings about it.
Aracelli: Yes, let's do that. I can take the iPad into the kitchen and ask the kids if they want a snack.
Therapist: Are you aware of any parts objecting right now?
Aracelli: Yeah, the Bossy Mom is saying, "Don't do it! They'll get sick and it'll be your fault!"
Therapist: And how do you respond?
Aracelli: Well, I know that's not true.

Therapist: See if you can let her feel your confidence and ask her allow you to make the call.
Aracelli: OK, she doesn't love it but she is not taking over.
Therapist: See if any other parts have anything to say.
Aracelli: There's the part that gets really frustrated with OCD, and it is rooting for me, but I also notice that I feel intimidated by the bossy part.... Usually that part feels like me. It's how I mostly respond, but right now I can see it as separate and it is daunting.
Therapist: What do you want to say to the part of you who is intimidated by the bossy one?
Aracelli: I let it know I'm here, and I've got this and it seems OK now... I think I want to just go try this. I can hear them in the kitchen. I want to give them the watermelon.
Therapist: OK, let's go.

Aracelli is wearing earbuds so I'm able to coach her as she offers the fruit to her kids. (The family knows me and understands what we're doing.) Aracelli and I talk about parts that come up as she watches her children eat the fruit. First, a part wanted to ask her husband for reassurance, so she asked that one to just sit back. Then a shaky, scared feeling came up and she was able to open her heart to that young part and let her know that she's not alone. And as the Bossy Mom saw that Aracelli was in charge of the situation and able to be with the anxious feelings, she quieted down, too. As we stayed there and watched the kids eat the fruit, then run off to play, Aracelli commented that it was the first time she'd been able to watch these parts come and go and not be taken over by them. She had gutted it out before in traditional ERP attempts but had never had this kind of experience: getting to know the parts of herself who object while allowing the thoughts and feelings to come and go with compassion, in a Self-led way.

After this session, Aracelli began to practice on her own. She let her kids eat the lunch served at their summer camp, popcorn and cookies from the bake sale. They even ate store-bought macaroni salad and worked up to the scariest food of all for her: sushi. Each time she encountered a new trigger situation, Aracelli took herself through a similar experience as above. She would be aware of the obsession, connect with her sense of Self, and allow the anxiety feeling to arise but not overtake her. She would talk to the compulsive firefighters in her mind, helping them to unblend and pause as she demonstrated to herself and her parts that she could handle the situation even if she had some anxious feelings.

Each time Aracelli managed to accomplish something that she previously was unable to even consider, her parts gained more trust, and she experienced more confidence. Greater courage, one of the 8 C's, made it easier for her to take the next risk that felt important to her. She slowly developed a sense of security that made it OK to not always "feel safe." Engaging in these exposures as more relational encounters with her parts became a welcome challenge for Aracelli, who was no longer as concerned with getting rid of the intrusive thoughts. These popup thoughts became familiar and less threatening once she took a pragmatic approach and changed her behaviors. She discovered she didn't have to wait until something felt safe to give it a try.

Justin's Decision to Reengage with Life

Some clients may prefer to see life itself as an exposure and not purposefully engage in intentional exposures—and that works too. Still, it's often helpful if therapists facilitate the first experiment so we can lend our Self-energy to the experience and help parts trust that reengaging in valued life activities might not be as difficult as anticipated.

Once Justin had enough access to Self to take a compassionate and curious stance toward his exiled parts he became more willing to accept their feelings without his OC protectors mediating the exchange. He successfully updated his protectors, letting them know he was able to be with fear and disgust without their interference. But, as in many cases, his protectors did not acknowledge the change right away. Because he had decided that he wanted to engage in life activities that he had avoided for many years, it became clear that he needed to negotiate with his parts.

Justin: I have an opportunity to move up at work but if I do, I'll have to go into the office and I can't be doing all my rituals or commandeer a bathroom for hours.
Therapist: Check inside and see what comes up as you think about doing that.
Justin: I think I could do it—but the Scout is still telling me that he'll pay attention to absolutely everything.
Therapist: What else do you hear inside?
Justin: I hear a part warning me that it'll do whatever it has to do if the part with all the dread takes over.
Therapist: How do you want to answer?
Justin: I appreciate the dedication, but I want my life back. If I feel that dread, I know I'll survive. I can invite the one that feels the fear and take care of it. Then I'll wash like everyone else does.
Therapist: How is the Scout doing?
Justin: Wow—as I say all that, other parts of me seem relieved. It's so excruciating to have to do all those rituals. I really don't want to do them anymore. The Scout stopped pacing for now, but he isn't going to go away.

Therapist: How do you feel about that?
Justin: I'm OK with it right now, but I think I might practice before I spend a whole day at work.

Once Justin had been able to work through the trauma that his OC parts had organized around, he regained a desire to engage in life and this became the motivation to face his feared triggers. At first, he needed to experience the confidence-boosting exposures in discrete increments—then he decided to let life itself be his exposure. He committed to noticing his compulsive firefighters when they stepped up and to relating to them differently, from Self. As he engaged in activities that took him further from home for longer periods of time, he found himself in situations where he had to do things that would previously have involved painstaking compulsions that he couldn't do without calling a great deal of attention to himself. Now that he had access to Self and a better relationship with his protectors, he was able to face these situations when they came up with a sense of freedom and letting go.

Step 4: Bringing It All Together

As Stage Three moves toward completion, we offer OC protectors the opportunity to find their new role or develop their capacity for moderation through the patience and kindness of Self-led practice. The more clients begin to engage in the previously avoided activities of life, the more opportunities OC protectors have to watch the Self in action. This builds on and reinforces their confidence in Self. Such experiments allow clients to deepen the connection with their authentic desires and experience the difference between a true Self and an obsessional manager who tells stories. This ability to differentiate helps clients more easily make the shift to trusting Self in all areas of life—those that typically trigger OCD and those that don't. As with the exile in Stage Two, we extend an invitation to OC protectors to welcome qualities and lost capacities, and we offer our appreciation to all parts who participated or allowed the work to happen.

Scott, who struggled with uncertainty and a Quality Control part who would tolerate no moral ambiguity, found some activities more difficult than others. Still, he remained able to welcome uncertainty, allowing his courageous Self to take the lead and make choices. He found that having compassion for all of his parts allowed them to be more flexible.

Aracelli, when connected with Self's confidence and clarity, found that her Bossy Mom let go of a lot of fear, and she was able to focus her attention on her desire to be a good mother. Paying attention to the value and vitality she found in that helped her protectors show up in a more balanced manner and with a less critical inner dialogue. She learned to appreciate the alert quality of the part she came to call her Good Enough Mom protector and was able to direct it in more creative ways that gave her a sense of accomplishment.

Justin was able to relax a little more once we helped the exiled part that was motivating his Scout and helped the protector release some of the weight of his over-valued responsibility. By engaging in life as it came, and being with the feelings as they came up, Justin helped the previously vigilant Scout learn to trust. By gradually encountering the situations he had avoided while unblending and letting Self take the lead, Justin could warmly acknowledge parts with fears and move toward a bigger life rather than avoiding it.

Throughout this stage, in varying ways, we enlist the principles of accepting uncertainty and unblending or disengaging from intrusive thoughts presenting as obsessional managers, and we reduce over-responsibility by unburdening OC protectors. We help clients rehearse and then practice gradually confronting feared situations without engaging in compulsions, and we help the more Self-led system learn to compassionately be with and tolerate doubt and ambiguity—rather than allowing protectors to remediate vulnerable feelings by seeking perfect certainty. Able to feel the compassionate presence of Self, clients report an inner sense of being their own secure attachment figure, and that slowly replaces a protector-driven need for safety and ultimately the need for the therapeutic structure.

Stage Three anchors awareness in the capacities that protectors had before they became extreme by facilitating an invitation to them to perform their previous, more balanced roles, allowing them to function in the way they were intended to. It's as if the OC protectors, by letting go of their extreme roles, shed their identities as OC parts and rejoin the whole, more integrated system of parts. Using the metaphor of spaciousness, clients find that their parts are still there, but there's plenty of space internally for those with differing thoughts and feelings to coexist. In the context of Self, parts are present but do not crowd our awareness.

Self-led ERP spends considerable time with the protective subsystem after the encounter and healing steps with exiles because it takes time and experience for the client to be able to replace the highly effective, short-term efforts of the OC protectors with more transformative behaviors. OC protectors are so strong, intractable, and Self-like because they've long been reinforced, sometimes for many years, before they've become distressingly counterproductive. Also, their dual connection to both neurobiology and exiles builds an intricate web of relationships that can be difficult to unravel. Improving the Self-to-protector relationships allows learning from experiences to build new connections that generalize and become more reliable over time.

With Self-leadership as the overarching goal, Self-led ERP is one method of using IFS for OCD. It integrates the benefits of the gold-standard, evidence-based, tried-and-true treatment approach for OCD with the relational and constraint-relieving approach of IFS. The intentional encounter with an exile in which Self is available and present with the part, willing to feel its burdens, beliefs, and stuck feelings, functions in the same way as a well-executed exposure in ERP. However, in the spirit of IFS, we do not *prevent* OC protectors from doing their jobs; instead, we befriend them so they can learn to trust Self. When protectors register that they are being acknowledged, they are more willing to hold back on their OC activity for long enough to see that it's possible, with Self in the lead, for the intensity of the feelings carried by exiles to be felt until they are healed or dissipate on their own without the protectors' intervention. The result is that the client's whole system is more balanced and secure, even in the face of challenges.

The three cases that we followed on this journey represent just a few of the ways in which clients can benefit from the addition of IFS to OCD treatment. They each tried evidence-based treatment and either plateaued, got stuck, or opted out. Adding IFS, but an OCD-informed IFS, provided another language and stance from which to engage with the escalating OC processes. Clients may particularly benefit from this approach when co-occurring diagnoses such as trauma, addiction, and eating disorders complicate OCD treatment. Others find it valuable at the end of treatment to work through residual interpersonal issues without triggering OC cycles. IFS for OCD is a compassionate approach to help clients with OCD to engage more fully in evidence-based OCD treatments such as ERP, ACT, and I-CBT or to use empirically supported processes and principles in a different way. This powerful integration of therapeutic modalities empowers clients to not only reduce their symptoms of OCD but also to know themselves more deeply, so they can live with more courage, creativity, and connection.

References

Anderson, F. G., Sweezy, M., & Schwartz, R. C. (2017). *Internal family systems skills training manual: Trauma-informed treatment for anxiety, depression, PTSD & substance abuse*. PESI Publishing & Media.

Hayes, S. C., Strosahl, K., & Wilson, K. G. (2003). *Acceptance and commitment therapy: An experiential approach to behavior change* (Paperback ed.). Guilford Press.

O'Connor, K., & Aardema, F. (2013). *Clinician's handbook for obsessive-compulsive disorder: Inference-based therapy*. Wiley-Blackwell.

Afterword

As we conclude this journey through the integration of Internal Family Systems (IFS) therapy and evidence-based treatments for obsessive-compulsive disorder (OCD), it seems fitting to reflect on both the evolution that brought us here and the path that lies ahead.

The development of IFS for OCD and Self-led ERP, my reframing of exposure and response prevention therapy, represents not just another therapeutic technique—it embodies a philosophical shift in how we help our clients. For too long, the field has been divided between approaches that prioritize symptom reduction and those that emphasize healing. This division has often, especially with OCD, forced clinicians to choose between effectiveness and compassion, between evidence-based protocols and relational depth.

What I have attempted to offer in these pages is a bridge between worlds that need not remain separate. The integration of IFS with established OCD treatments honors both the research that addresses the neurobiological realities of the disorder, and its treatment, and the relational wisdom of the mindfulness-based traditions, and their awareness of Self. It recognizes that while intrusive thoughts may arise from brain circuitry beyond conscious control, our relationship with these experiences—and the parts of us that respond to them—can be transformed.

Those who suffer from OCD know all too well the experience of feeling hijacked by their own minds, of being simultaneously the one who fears and the one who tries desperately to control that fear. The Self-led ERP approach offers a new possibility: the capacity to witness both the obsessional managers and compulsive firefighters from a place of compassionate curiosity, to understand their protective intentions while gently guiding them toward less extreme roles.

For clinicians, this integration invites a more flexible therapeutic stance. Rather than positioning ourselves as experts directing clients through prescribed exposures, we become companions in exploration, helping them encounter their exiled parts to access their own healing capacity. We need not abandon the proven mechanisms that make ERP effective but we can deliver this powerful medicine in a form that clients find more meaningful and sustainable.

The cases presented throughout this book represent real people with real struggles, though details have been changed and compiled to protect confidentiality. Their journeys remind us that recovery from OCD is rarely linear or complete. The neurobiological vulnerability that contributes to OCD may remain, occasionally generating intrusive thoughts or urges even after successful treatment. But with Self-leadership established, these experiences need not trigger the same intensity of distress or cycles of obsession and compulsion.

As this approach continues to develop, we welcome further refinement, dialogue, and ultimately, some solid research. The integration presented here is not meant to be the final word, but rather an invitation to a conversation about how we might better serve those struggling with OCD. It is my hope that clinicians from various theoretical orientations will find something valuable in these pages—whether you are an IFS therapist seeking to work more effectively with OCD or an OCD specialist interested in incorporating parts-work into your practice.

Ultimately, the measure of any therapeutic approach lies not in its theoretical elegance but in its capacity to alleviate suffering and promote flourishing. As you apply these principles and techniques in your own practice, I encourage you to hold both aims in mind: Helping clients find relief from debilitating symptoms while also supporting their journey toward a more harmonious, balanced, and secure relationship with all parts of themselves.

The path of healing is rarely straight, but it need not be walked alone. I hope that this integration serves as one more light illuminating the way toward greater Self-leadership for both clinicians and those they serve.

Index

Note: *Italic* page numbers refer to figures and page numbers followed by "n" denote endnotes.

Aardema, F. 77
abject terror 53
acceptance 24, 71, 76, 114–115, 117, 128, 161, 169, 170, 172–173, 182, 185
acceptance and commitment therapy (ACT) 75–76, 81, 115, 119, 122, 129–131, 168n1, 187
alarm systems 42, 45, 92–93, 107
alliances 15–16, 34, 91, 95, 103, 109–111, 114
American Psychiatric Association 41, 59; *Diagnostic and Statistical Manual of Mental Disorders, Fifth Edition* 41, 58–59
anxiety disorder 1, 51
assessments: initial 66–67; of OCD 58–61
attention-deficit/ hyperactivity disorder (ADHD) 57

befriending 24–28, 119–125; principles at work in 124–125
behavioral rituals 46, 62
blending 90, 96, 120–122, 139, 146
brain–body system 41, 190
burden 16–17, 21, 31–33, 78–79, 88, 90–94, 96, 99–101, 105, 107–108, 111, 118, 126, 128–129, 137, 141, 143, 146, 163–164, 169–172, 178, 180–186, 188–190

cognitive behavioral therapy (CBT) 77, 88, 123
cognitive therapy 88

committed action 76
compulsions 42, 44–47
compulsive firefighter 91, 93–94, 98, 100, 103–107, 109–113, 118, 123, 131, 138, 144, 154–155, 161, 164, 166, 171, 178, 185, 187, 189, 197
conference table and variations 34–35
contamination-focused obsessions 62–63, 99
Craske, Michelle 73

danger learning 73
decentering 119–120, 122–123
defusion 76, 120, 122–123; from self as content 122; unblending to differentiate parts 122
Diagnostic and Statistical Manual of Mental Disorders, Fifth Edition (American Psychiatric Association) 41, 58–59
direct access 35–36
do over 175–179
dynamic OC cycle 107–109, *107*

ego-dystonic 44, 51
8 C's 10, 12, 24, 26–28, 89, 123, 141, 153, 155, 159, 195, 197
emotional contamination 62
emotional processing theory (EPT) 71
emotion regulation 22, 119–120, 123–124
encountering/unburdening exiles 169–184
engaging: OC protectors 129–131; principles at work in 129–131

evidence-based psychotherapeutic interventions 70
evidence-based treatment options 67, 69–82; experience as umbrella concept 74–79; exposure as mechanism of healing 70–74; limitations of 79–81; for OCD 69–82; refining current approaches and integrating IFS 81–82
expectancy violation 73, 80–81, 130, 171
experience as umbrella concept 74–79
experience-near approach 43, 62
experimenting to access Self 154
explicit direct access 36
exposure: as mechanism of healing 70–74; witnessing exile from Self 127
exposure and response prevention (ERP) therapy 1–3, 69, 88, 115, 120–122
exposure-based interventions: habituation explanation 71–72; inhibitory learning theory explanation 73–74
exposure-based treatments 70
external constraints 141
externalizing methods for facilitating unblending 34

family accommodation (FA) 48
family systems therapy 9
faulty inference 77
Feared Possible Self (FPS) 78, 127–128
firefighter–OC subsystem polarizations 112–113
firefighters 17–19, 91, 93–94, 98, 100, 103–107, 109–113, 118, 123, 131, 138, 144, 154–155, 161, 164, 166, 171, 178, 185, 187, 189, 197
5 P's 22
Foa, E. B. 71, 96–97

going inside process 25–28

habituation 71–74; habituation explanation 71–72
harm-focused obsessions 63–64
healing: exposure as mechanism of 70–74; steps 29–33
Hershfield, Jon 127
hierarchies between systems 113–114

IFS-informed OCD assessment 137–148; applying 139–141; background 141–142; benefits of 147–148; level of insight 146; obsessions and compulsions 142–144; prompts and triggers 145; relevant history 141–142; severity of symptoms 144–145; symptoms of OCD 142–144
IFS therapists: knowing internal systems 22–23; qualities of 21–23
IFS therapy: art of 36; attending to the needs of exiles 29–33; BeFriend 28; building trust with protectors 24–28; direct access 35–36; feel toward 27–28; find 27; flesh out 27; focus on 27; goals of 19; healing steps 29–33; identify fears 28; IFS therapist 21–23; insight 35; methods used in 33–36; process and methods of 21–37; protector interactions and relationships 33–35; re-establishing trust 29–33; unblending and befriending 24–28
implicit direct access 36
inference-based cognitive behavioral therapy (I-CBT) 77–79, 99, 125, 127, 129, 131, 168n1, 187
inferential confusion 77–79, 119–120, 125, 131
inhibitory learning theory (ILT) 73–74, 130
initial assessments 66–67
integrating: and appreciation 32–33; new relationships 130; OC protectors 129–131; principles at work in 129–131
internal constraints 141
Internal Family Systems (IFS) 3–5, 9–19, 21, 43, 51, 57–58, 69, 87, 89, 137, 149, 185; alliances and polarizations 15–16; befriending 119–125; burdens and exiles 16–17; compulsive firefighters 98; conceptualization of OCD 87–101; different about for OCD 91–94; exiles 99–100; goals of IFS therapy 19; integrated, principles-driven approach 115–117; language of 89–90; managers and firefighters 17–19; multiplicity of mind 10–12; neurobiological factors 92–93; obsessional managers 96–98; OC

cycle 93–94; and OCD cycle 103–114; proactive managers 17–18; processes at work in IFS for OCD 119; protectors' burdens and OCD system 100–101; reactive firefighters 18–19; reconnecting with protectors 128–131; refining current approaches and integrating 81–82; Self and its resources 10; Self-leadership 12–13, 94–95; Stage One 119–125; Stage Three 128–131; Stage Two 125–128; three stages of IFS for OCD 117–119; unblending 13–15, 119–125; useful for clients with OCD 115–132; vulnerable parts and protective parts 16; witnessing and retrieval 125–128
intolerance of uncertainty–focused obsessions 65–66
invitation 32
in vivo 167, 172
Is Fred in the Refrigerator? (Nicely) 169

Kozak, M. J. 71

Lebois, L. A. M. 123

magical obsessions 65
manager–OC subsystem polarizations 111–112
managers 17–19
mapping parts 34
mental health syndromes 41
mental rituals 46, 62, 98, 104
mindfulness 76–77, 127; decentering and 122–123; and self-compassion based exposure 127; techniques 75, 77; unblending to shift perspectives 122–123
mindfulness-informed approaches 88
multiplicity of mind 4, 10–12

Nicely, Shala 169; *Is Fred in the Refrigerator?* 169

obsessional doubt 77, 78, 125, 131, 147, 153, 166
obsessional manager 91–94, 96–98, 100–101, 103–109, 111–113, 118, 120–121, 125, 131, 138, 145, 154–155, 161, 164, 167, 172, 183, 185
obsessional sequence 78

obsessional story 78
obsessions 42, 44–45
obsessive-compulsive (OC) cycle 93–94, 103, *107*; adaptations of IFS tools for unblending 153–154; alliances within the OC subsystem 110; dynamics of *106*, 106–108, *107*; hierarchies between systems 113–114; polarizations with the outer system 110–113; protector interactions 109–114
obsessive-compulsive disorder (OCD) 1–4, 41, 66, 87, 96, *106*, 110, 115, 137, 143, 149, 150; assessment of OCD 58–61; background and relevant history 59; brief history of 41–44; case examples 52–53; clinical applications 61; compulsions 45–47; contamination-focused obsessions 62–63; described 51; different about IFS for 91–94; differentiating 49–51; evidence-based treatment options for 69–82; exiles carry themes and burdens of uncertainty 99–100; family accommodation 48; harm-focused obsessions 63–64; IFS conceptualization of 87–101; IFS-informed assessment of 137–148; IFS useful for clients with 115–132; increasing awareness about 57–58; initial assessments 66–67; intolerance of uncertainty-focused obsessions 65–66; language of IFS for 89–90; level of insight 60–61; obsessions 44–45; OCD cycle 47–48; processes at work in IFS for 119; prompts and triggers 60; rightness, symmetry, and order-focused obsessions 64; Self-leadership and 94–95; severity of symptoms 60; subtypes of OCD 61–66; symptoms of 59–60; three stages of IFS for 117–119; unacceptable or taboo thoughts–focused obsessions 64–65
obsessive-compulsive (OC) subsystem 149
OCD Bubble 127–128
OCD cycle: role of family accommodation in maintaining 48; through an IFS lens 103–114

OC exiles 16–17, 21, 118, 164–167, 169–184; encountering an exile is exposure 170–172; encountering the exile 174–179; retrieval 179–180; unburdening and invitation 180–183
OC firefighter 90, 112, 142, 168
OC manager 90, 91, 99, 101, 103, 105, 107, 121, 140, 142, 144, 153, 165
O'Connor, K. 77–78
OC protectors: contracting with 154; engaging 129–131; integrating 129–131; updating 129–131
OC subsystem 4, 89, 90, 92–93, 95, 98, 100, 103–114, 120, 126, 138–141, 144, 148, 152, 154, 164–166, 170–172, 174
order-focused obsessions 64

Pediatric Acute-Onset Neuropsychiatric Syndrome (PANS) 41
Pediatric Autoimmune Neuropsychiatric Disorder Associated with Strep (PANDAS) 41
pedophilia-themed obsessions 63
persistent firefighters 166–167
polarizations 15–16; firefighter-OC subsystem 112–113; manager-OC subsystem 111–112; with the outer system 110–113
proactive manager 17–18, 90
processes: of IFS therapy 21–37; at work in IFS for OCD 119
prompts and triggers 60
protective parts 16
protector interactions and relationships 33–35, 109–114
protector parts and the Self 24
protectors 4, 66, 96, 143, 150; acceptance and willingness 130; and accessing Self 149–168; building trust with 24–28; burdens fuel the OCD system 100–101; contracting with 154; helping OC protectors unblend 154–166; helping system-wide protectors unblend 151–153; integrating the new relationships 130; negotiating permission to go to the exiles 166–167; OC adaptations of IFS tools for unblending 153–154; reconnecting with 128–131, 185–201; unblending and befriending 24–28; update, engage, and integrate 129–131; updating about the encounter 130
psychological disorder 12
PTSD symptom reduction 119
purely obsessional OCD 44

Quinlan, Kimberley 125

reactive firefighters 18–19
reality sensing 131
real Self 131
reappraisal 123
reasoning behind obsessional doubt 125
reassurance seeking 1, 46, 62, 165; reassurance-seeking compulsions 63
rehearsing self-leadership 131
religious scrupulosity 64
retrieval 31, 127–128; Internal Family Systems (IFS) 125–128; principles at work in 127–128
rightness, and OCD 64

safety learning 73, 74, 129–130
Schwartz, Richard 9–11, 13, 16, 19
Seif, M. N. 117
Self: and protector parts 24; resources of 10; witnessing the exile from 127
Self-as-context 76
self-compassion 77, 124–125
self compassion–based exposure therapy 76–77, 127
Self Compassion Workbook for ERP 125
self-destructive behaviors 18
Self-energy 12, 21, 23–27, 36, 121, 153–154, 159, 163, 182, 194
self-harm ideation 65
Self-leadership 12–13, 73, 79, 91, 94–95, 107, 116–117, 120, 129, 131, 149, 150, 168, 175, 182, 185, 187, 191
Self-led exposure and response prevention (Self-led ERP) 137–138, 140, 149–151, 153, 155, 163, 166, 168, 168n1, 169–170, 185, 189, 194, 201
Self-led regulation 123

self-processing 123
self-related processing 123
Self-to-part relationships 21, 29, 61, 116, 125, 130, 146, 195
sexual behaviors 64
sexuality-focused obsessions 99
sexual obsessions 65
6 F's 23, 26, 28, 35, 115, 154–155
subjective units of distress (SUDs) 72
Sweezy, Martha 119, 126
symmetry, and OCD 64
Szymanksi, Jeff 81

thought-thought fusion 47, 93, 104
trailheads 27, 155–156
treatment-interfering behaviors 2
trust: building with protectors 24–28; do over 30–31; integration and appreciation 32–33; invitation 32; re-establishing 29–33; retrieval 31; unblending and befriending 24–28; unburdening 31–32; witnessing 30

unacceptable/taboo thoughts–focused obsessions 64–65
unblending 24–28, 119–125; to differentiate parts 122; ERP 120–122; externalizing methods for facilitating 34; OC adaptations of IFS tools for 153–154; from parts 13–15; principles at work in 120–123; for self-led regulation 123; to shift perspectives 122–123; using experiments to facilitate 120–122
unburdening 31–32, 127–128
uncertainty-focused obsessions 61
updating: OC protectors 129–131; principles at work in 129–131

validated exposure approaches 75
violence-focused obsessions 99
vulnerable parts 16
Vulnerable Self Theme 78

Winston, S. M. 117
witnessing 30, 174–179; the exile from self 127; Internal Family Systems (IFS) 125–128; mindfulness and self-compassion based exposure 127; principles at work in 127–128
World Health Organization 42

Yale-Brown Obsessive-Compulsive Scale 60